Geriatric Mental Health Ethics

Shane S. Bush, PhD, ABPP, ABPN, is the director of Long Island Neuropsychology, P.C., and is a clinical assistant professor in the Department of Psychiatry and Behavioral Science, State University of New York at Stony Brook School of Medicine. He is board certified in clinical neuropsychology and rehabilitation psychology by the American Board of Professional Psychology, and is board certified in neuropsychology by the American Board of Professional Neuropsychology. He is a fellow of the American Psychological Association's Divisions of Neuropsychology, Rehabilitation Psychology, and Adult Development and Aging and is a fellow of the National Academy of Neuropsychology. He is an editorial board member of *The Clinical Neuropsychologist, Applied Neuropsychology, Archives of Clinical Neuropsychology*, and *Journal of Head Trauma Rehabilitation*. He has published five books and two special journal issues on ethical issues and one book on geriatric neuropsychology. He has also published articles, chapters, and position papers on ethical and professional issues, and has presented on professional ethics at national conferences.

Geriatric Mental Health Ethics

A Casebook

SHANE S. BUSH, PhD, ABPP, ABPN

SPRINGER PUBLISHING COMPANY

New York

Springer Publishing Company, LLC
11 West 42nd Street
New York, NY 10036
www.springerpub.com

Acquisitions Editor: Philip Laughlin
Project Manager: Cindy Fullerton
Cover Design: Joanne E. Honigman
Composition: Aptara Inc.

08 09 10 11 12/5 4 3 2 1

Library of Congress Cataloging-in-Publication Data
Bush, Shane S., 1965–
    Geriatric mental health ethics : a casebook / Shane S. Bush.
        p. ; cm.
    Includes bibliographical references and index.
    ISBN 978-0-8261-0319-2 (alk. paper)
1. Geriatric psychiatry–Moral and ethical aspects–Case studies.   2. Older people
Case studies–Mental health services–Moral and ethical aspects   I. Title.
    [DNLM: 1. Mental Health Services–ethics.   2. Aged.   3. Ethics, Professional.
4. Health Services for the Aged–ethics.   5. Mental Disorders–therapy.
WM 30 B9784g 2009]
    RC451.4.A5B84 2009
    174.2′9689—dc22

                                                                              2008036376

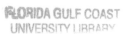

To the older adults in my personal and professional lives who have shared their experiences and, through their present, have given me glimpses into both the past and the future. I hope that I provided something of value in return.
And
To Dana, Sarah, and Megan—always.

Contents

Foreword

As this thoughtful and informative volume on the ethical/legal implications of geriatric mental health treatment is being written, nearly 8,000 U.S. residents are turning 60 each day (www.census.gov/ipc/www/usinterimproj/). Just as the demographics are mandating an adequately trained mental health workforce to address this burgeoning population, the Institute of Medicine (IOM) released on April 14, 2008 the "Retooling for an Aging America: Building the Health Care Workforce" (www.iom.edu/CMS/3809/40113/53452.aspx). This report recommends that the workforce demonstrate competency in the care of older adults as a requirement for licensure and certification. It also calls on employers and regulators to expand the roles of individuals who care for older adults with complex clinical needs at different levels of the health care system beyond the traditional scope of medical practice. The author's teaching goal of increased competence in ethical decision making and practice associated with the complexity of treating older mental health patients is certainly consistent with the IOM's mandate and is a welcome tool in the preparation of the future mental health workforce.

Dr. Bush has written this book from an interdisciplinary and clinically based approach. Challenging learning experiences are presented at the conclusion of each chapter, and a dozen diverse case studies guide the reader/learner through the "4 A's" of ethical decision making and practice. Using an educational approach, the reader is prepared to learn how to *Anticipate* and prepare for the ethical issues inherent in geriatric mental health, cautioned so as to *Avoid* the pitfalls of ethical dilemmas, instructed how to develop a strategy to *Address* the ethical challenges, and inspired to *Aspire* to even higher standards of ethical decision making and practice.

As a geriatric psychiatrist, I have been faced with many of the dilemmas posed in this casebook. The knowledge and use of professional ethical codes, laws, practice guidelines, and colleagues' expertise are invaluable in my day-to-day practice. The decision-making model proposed by Dr. Bush is a construct that can be used by any mental health professional and in all treatment settings. Dr. Bush asks in his conclusion if we, as mental health professionals, are ready for the task of facing this exciting and complex challenge of treatment of the aging in this country. After reading this innovative casebook, I am inspired to face these challenges with a new perspective and encourage others along the way to be better advocates and clinicians.

Lory Bright-Long, MD, CMD
Clinical Assistant Professor, Department of Psychiatry &
Behavioral Sciences, Stony Brook University School of Medicine
Geropsychiatry Consultant, Long Island State Veterans Home
Medical Director, Maria Regina Residence

Introduction

Providing mental health services to older adults can be as ethically challenging as it is personally rewarding. Like clinical challenges, ethical dilemmas often emerge in unique and unexpected ways. Yet, I wonder if we, as mental health professionals, are as prepared to handle ethical dilemmas as we are clinical challenges? I suspect that the vast majority of us can describe the theoretical model or models upon which we rely in our clinical decision making with older adults. However, how many of us can describe *any* ethical decision-making model, let alone one that we regularly use to resolve ethical challenges in our work with older adults? Similarly, I imagine that most of us can name at least a few professional references to which we can turn to find answers to clinical questions. But, other than the ethics code of our own discipline, how many professional references can we name that provide direction and answers for our ethical challenges?

A primary ethical responsibility is professional competence, from both clinical and ethical perspectives. Like clinical competence, ethical competence requires us to challenge ourselves and each other on an ongoing basis to explore the boundaries of our ethical knowledge and confront and expand those boundaries. A primary goal of this book is to challenge you, the reader, to question your own ethical competence and to use the information and decision-making model presented in the book to reinforce and expand the boundaries of your ethical competence; writing the book has helped do so for me.

The primary purposes of this casebook are to (a) describe ethical challenges commonly encountered by mental health professionals who serve the elderly, (b) review resources available for ethical decision making, (c) present an ethical decision-making model, and (d) demonstrate the application of the ethical decision-making model through clinical cases. To achieve these goals, an emphasis is placed on identifying the similarities and clarifying the differences among clinical, ethical, legal, and professional contributions to complex cases. The information presented in this book is intended to apply across mental health contexts and disciplines. Advanced consideration of ethical issues that arise during the practice of geriatric mental health care, and options for addressing such issues, prepares clinicians to practice in a manner that advances the welfare of patients, families, and other consumers of mental health services.

Much of the information in this book builds on my previous writings and focuses those prior ideas and ethical explorations onto the world of geriatric mental health. In the presentation of case vignettes, the ethics codes and resources that are considered most relevant to the specific professional discipline presented in the vignette are relied upon for the analysis of the ethical issues and challenges. For example, in case vignettes that involve social workers, the Code of Ethics of the National Association of Social Workers (1996) is emphasized, although other relevant resources may be included as well. Similarly, the ethics codes of other mental health disciplines are emphasized in the analysis of case vignettes that involve those disciplines. However, the potential value of "ethical cross-training" (Bush, 2008) cannot be overstated.

This book could not have been written without the direct and indirect assistance of many friends and colleagues. Among those who most directly influenced my thinking about ethical issues in geriatric mental health are Drs. Frank Cervo and Lory Bright-Long. Through long discussions at the Long Island State Veterans Home at Stony Brook University, we examined ethical challenges related to patients/residents and their families, professional behavior, and policy issues. Although we did not resolve all of the problems, I believe we sparked an ongoing commitment to try, and I am grateful to Drs. Cervo and Bright-Long for it. I also want to thank my good friend and frequent collaborator, Dr. Tom Martin, for our exchanges of thoughts and manuscripts on ethical issues in geriatric neuropsychology. Additionally, I want to extend my appreciation once again to Drs. Jerry Sweet and Joel Morgan for encouraging me to begin this journey of writing/editing books on ethics some 8 years and seven books ago. Finally, I want to thank Springer Publisher Company and acquisitions editor Philip Laughlin for all of the assistance, support, and patience needed to complete a project that I hope ultimately helps to improve the lives of older adults receiving mental health services.

1 Developmental Considerations

The population of older adults in the U.S. is growing rapidly, with a corresponding increase in the number of older adults evaluated and treated by mental health professionals. It is anticipated that approximately 71.5 million people will be over the age of 65 in the United States by the year 2030 (Federal Interagency Forum on Aging-Related Statistics, 2006). Additionally, it has been predicted that the number of individuals who are 85 years of age and older will double, and the number of individuals who are 100 or older will triple.

The transition into late adulthood, like other developmental transitions, is associated with physical and psychosocial changes, some advantageous and others adverse. Late adulthood, like other stages of the life cycle, offers opportunities for growth and change that enrich life. The shift in biomedical and social sciences in recent years from an illness and disease–oriented model of aging toward a more adaptive model of health and wellness reflects the positive aspects of older adulthood (Beckingham & Watts, 1995; Bowling, 1993; Kaplan & Strawbridge, 1994; Knight, 2004; Myers, 1992). However, aging, like other life transitions, includes potential threats to successful adjustment (Coleman, 1992; Erikson, 1982).

Compared to earlier developmental stages, a primary challenge associated with late adulthood involves confronting loss (Myers, 1999; Waters & Goodman, 1990). Losses in the areas of sensory and motor abilities, cognitive functioning, social roles, financial resources, and long-term relationships are more common for older adults. Such losses may be accompanied by negative emotional changes (Erikson, 1963; Erikson, Erikson, & Kivnick, 1986; Lebowitz et al., 1997), as well as decreased resources for coping with the losses.

In addition to confronting loss, medical problems, physical pain, and medication usage occur with greater frequency for older adults. Approximately 80% of older adults have at least one chronic health problem, and about 50% of older adults have at least two chronic health problems (He, Sengupta, Velkoff, & DeBarros, 2005). Additionally, approximately 20% of older adults experience chronic disabilities, and 18% of men and 32% of women are unable to perform at least one basic physical function (Federal Interagency Forum on Aging-Related Statistics, 2006). These physical and psychosocial changes may result in increased dependence on others for assistance with daily tasks and decisions that were previously completed independently. Decreased autonomy in later adulthood can be associated with a host of emotional reactions, for both those with and without prior mental health needs. With depressive symptoms alone affecting approximately 15% of community-dwelling older adults and up to 25% of those in nursing homes (He et al., 2005), the need for competent mental health professionals to evaluate and treat older adults and their family members has never been greater, and it will increase for the foreseeable future.

From a clinical perspective, the developmental changes of late life pose unique professional and ethical challenges for clinicians who work with older adults (Hays, 1999). Individual differences in aspects of maturity, specific physical and psychosocial difficulties, cohort differences, and contextual social and treatment settings must all be considered and appropriately integrated into evaluation and treatment methods and decisions (Knight, 2004).

Treatment context may be one of the most readily apparent and distinguishable aspects of geriatric mental health services. Older adults receive mental health services in multiple clinical and residential settings. Although older adults are commonly evaluated and treated by mental health professionals across the same medical and mental health care settings in which younger adult patients are encountered, such as hospitals, outpatient physical medicine and rehabilitation programs, mental health clinics, and private practices, they are encountered in greater numbers in some of those settings because of the increased health problems and unique stressors associated with aging. In addition, because of the increased prevalence of chronic health problems and cognitive decline associated with aging, as well as limited personal and family resources for managing decreased functional abilities in the home, older adults also frequently receive mental health services through adult day care programs, assisted living facilities, and skilled nursing facilities. Mental health practitioners are frequently involved as consultants or integral members of the professional staff in the care of registrants or residents in such settings.

Each of these settings affects the clinical issues of concern to the patient and the clinician, and the clinical issues may evolve as the patient transitions from one setting to another. For example, a 79-year-old man with a history of diabetes may present to a private practice following amputations of both legs with significant sorrow over the loss of his legs, regret over his poor management of his diabetes, and guilt over the burden that he has become to his wife. Nevertheless, he may maintain a sense of determination to learn to use his prosthetics and other assistive devices, so that he can do more for himself at home and relieve his wife of some of the burden. However, should he not achieve his goals and instead be forced to move into a skilled nursing facility, he may feel anger and resentment toward his wife for what he perceives to be abandonment, and his determination may be replaced by a sense of hopelessness and despair. This man's emotional reaction may also increase his wife's feelings of guilt and sadness. Such psychological and interpersonal dynamics are encountered with considerable regularity for mental health professionals who work with the elderly.

Collaboration with other mental health and medical professionals is often essential to the effective care of older adults. For example, in skilled nursing facilities, it is common for residents to have their mental health needs addressed by multiple professionals, as well as paraprofessionals and volunteers. Consider the case of a 93-year-old woman who was living independently when her sweater caught fire while she was cooking, causing multiple severe burns that required skin grafts and a lengthy period of hospitalization. Following medical stabilization, she was transferred to a skilled nursing facility for subacute rehabilitation, with the hope that she would eventually return to her home. However, as time passed and she continued to need assistance for some of her daily activities, it became apparent that she would not be going home, at which time she became depressed. Crying episodes and decreased appetite were first noticed by her certified nursing assistant (CNA), who reported it to the nurse on duty. The nurse confirmed the CNA's impression and reported the apparent depression to the attending primary medical doctor (PMD). The PMD ordered a psychiatry consultation, at which point an antidepressant medication was prescribed. A psychologist was consulted for psychotherapy, and the social worker on the unit provided additional emotional support and located a relative who was glad to begin visiting on a regular basis. Increased involvement in recreational activities and visits from a young volunteer helped complete the interdisciplinary approach to the alleviation of the woman's adjustment-related depression.

The extent and nature of family involvement also distinguish the mental health treatment of many older adults from that of younger patients. Although some older adults find themselves increasingly isolated and lonely, others experience increased involvement of family members, which may or may not be welcome. Important clinical and ethical considerations correspond to the varying degrees and quality of family involvement.

Learning Exercises

1. He, Sengupta, Velkoff, and DeBarros (2005) found that depressive symptoms affect approximately 15% of community-dwelling older adults and up to what percent of those in nursing homes?

a. 20%
b. 25%
c. 55%
d. 85%

2. Older adulthood inevitably includes which one of the following?

a. Dementia
b. Diabetes
c. Anxiety
d. Loss

3. True/False. Unfortunately, unlike all of the previous developmental stages, older adulthood does not offer opportunities for personal growth and changes that enrich life.

2 Ethical Principles and Resources

Ethical decision making requires clinicians ultimately to decide, "What should I do?" However, we must first determine, "What should I take into consideration" (Cooper, 2007). Many ethical and legal resources exist for review, consultation, and consideration during the ethical decision-making process. To best understand our ethics codes and other resources, it can be advantageous to review the values and biomedical ethical principles that underlie such resources.

Professional ethics in the United States reflect the common morality or values of Western societies. The ability of competent adults to make the decisions that govern their lives is one such value held by Western societies, and is considered a fundamental human right. Similarly, the ability to live peacefully, to receive an education, to have access to competent health care, and to be treated fairly by the government are all highly valued and expected in Western societies. Values such as these, which are shared by members of a society are, by extension, generally reflected in the medical and mental health professions of the society and underlie the ethical principles that guide professional behavior.

Ethical principles and standards are based on the shared values of a profession for the protection and promotion of the welfare of patients, the profession, and society. The ability of clinicians to understand and appreciate the values held by patients and other consumers and to use that knowledge to protect and promote patient and consumer welfare is essential to ethical and legal practice.

PRINCIPLE-BASED ETHICS

Multiple philosophical systems are relevant for ethical decision making in the practice of geriatric mental health (Knapp & VandeCreek, 2006; Mahowald, 1994). Such systems include virtue ethics, utilitarianism, deontological ethics, and principle-based ethics. These systems provide organization for the shared values or a common morality (Knapp & VandeCreek, 2006) of a society. As important components of the society, the mental health professions rely on such philosophical systems for the foundation of their ethics codes.

Principle-based ethics, developed nearly a century ago (Ross, 1930/1998), has gained popularity and fairly widespread acceptance among medical and mental health professionals in recent years (Beauchamp & Childress, 2001). The ethics codes of various health care and mental health organizations have been informed by or adopted principle-based ethics to guide the behavior of their members. This utilization of a common philosophical system allows for a familiarity and a common language between clinicians that facilitates interdisciplinary communication regarding ethical matters.

Beauchamp and Childress (2001) presented four core biomedical ethical principles: respect for autonomy, nonmaleficence, beneficence, and justice. Respect for autonomy refers to the right of competent patients to make the decisions that govern their lives, as long as those decisions do not negatively impact the rights of others. This principle departs from the paternalistic approach traditionally encountered in medicine, whereby health care professionals assume to know which medical decisions are in the patient's best interests and what interventions should be administered. Respect for patient autonomy is based on the premise that a competent, well-informed adult patient can choose to accept or decline examination or treatment options and should be included in the decision-making process.

The principle of nonmaleficence addresses the classic mandate to do no harm. Although this principle may initially seem obvious, determinations regarding what constitutes harm or which individual, organization, or system is owed such an obligation can be difficult to make in a given case. Beneficence as an ethical principle refers to a moral obligation to take action to advance the welfare of others. Beneficence encompasses the promotion of the rights and health of others, as well as defense of the rights of others and the prevention of harm.

Justice is the availability and provision of "fair, equitable, and appropriate treatment in light of what is due or owed to persons" (Beauchamp & Childress, 2001, p. 226). Two types or components of justice are described: distributive justice and formal justice. Distributive justice refers to the equitable distribution of health care or mental health resources. Formal justice refers to equal treatment for those who are equals and unequal treatment for those who are not equals. Challenges to the successful application of the principle of justice lie in defining what is equitable and determining which individuals or groups are equals. Mental health professionals must consider these questions in the unique contexts in which ethical problem-solving occurs.

Two additional moral principles have been proposed as applicable to mental health professionals: fidelity and general beneficence (Knapp & VandeCreek, 2006). Fidelity (Bersoff & Koeppl, 1993; Kitchener, 1984) refers to the obligation to be truthful and faithful, keep promises, and maintain loyalty. General beneficence (Knapp & VandeCreek, 2006) refers to the clinician's responsibility to the public at large (i.e., society). As an example, these authors describe the responsibility of psychologists to protect future consumers of psychological evaluation services by safeguarding the integrity of psychological tests.

In the context of geriatric medicine and long-term care, Feinsod and Wagner (2007) offered 10 ethical principles. With the biomedical ethical principles described by Beauchamp and Childress (2001) as an underlying foundation, the addition of more specific principles such as "futility of treatment," "truth telling," and "non-abandonment" further delineates the clinician's ethical and professional responsibilities.

With regard to the possible futility of treatment, it can be easy for clinicians in long-term care facilities to establish relationships with residents or provide treatments that reflect "friendly visits," and are perceived as such by the residents, more than mental health treatment per se. Although residents may appreciate such visits, the clinical value above what an untrained volunteer can provide may be difficult to discern at times. In such instances, clinicians have responsibility to review treatment goals, determine whether the goals are consistent with the patient's wishes and are clinically realistic, assess whether the treatment is beneficial, and modify or terminate treatment as appropriate (Feinsod & Wagner, 2007).

"Truth telling" refers to the clinician's duty to be honest with the patient rather than provide incomplete or inaccurate statements of encouragement (Feinsod & Wagner, 2007). Hiding behind medical terminology when discussing diagnosis and prognosis should be avoided. However, blatant honesty, even when conveyed as sensitively as possible, can be extremely painful. As with any bad news, when a physician or other clinician provides a patient with a truthful but negative assessment of her medical status or prognosis, it may be the responsibility of the mental health professional to help the patient process the new information.

The principle of "non-abandonment" addresses what is often a fine line between appropriate termination or transfer of treatment and the neglectful ending of a therapeutic relationship. Clinicians may become discouraged or frustrated with a patient or patient's family for many reasons, including a lack of compliance with treatment or other recommendations and challenging, threatening, seductive, or intrusive personality traits. Clinician's may end treatment relationships when reasonable time and resources have been provided to the patient or the proxy to facilitate an appropriate transition to another clinician (Feinsod & Wagner, 2007). When conflicts between clinicians and patients or proxies arise, it can be helpful and necessary to seek guidance or assistance from an ombudsman, ethics committee, Department of Health, and/or other appropriate persons or agencies.

General ethical principles provide valuable guidance in determining a good course of action, particularly when the ethical standards of a given ethics code do not provide the needed direction to resolve an ethical challenge, and when ethical standards within an ethics code conflict with each other or with jurisdictional laws. However, instances also arise in which these biomedical ethical principles conflict with each other. For example, respect for patient autonomy conflicts with beneficence or general beneficence when patients report an intention to harm themselves or others. Although in this example the relative importance of the principles is clear (i.e., beneficence takes precedence over autonomy), in other situations it is difficult to determine which principle must be given greater weight, leaving the clinician to make such judgments. In such instances, use of an ethical decision-making model can be particularly helpful.

ETHICS CODES

The professional organizations of each mental health profession have ethics codes that describe appropriate professional conduct (see Table 2.1). The ethics codes of the different disciplines vary somewhat in the degree to which they address specific or general behaviors or provide enforceable standards or aspirational principles. However, all of the ethics codes strive to present the shared values of their discipline. Because of the common morality of Western societies, considerable overlap occurs among the ethics codes of the mental health professions. Despite the overlap, however, each discipline offers unique contributions to mental health care, which reinforces the value of each code for helping clinicians to determine acceptable behaviors for their unique aspects of practice. For example, physicians and others with prescription privileges, or psychologists who administer standardized psychological or neurocognitive tests, will find aspects of these professional activities in their ethics codes and professional guidelines. Familiarity with the ethics codes of colleagues from different disciplines can be informative when considering ethical challenges and striving to better understand the values and motivations of clinicians whose roles overlap in the treatment of older adults.

Table 2.1

SELECTED MENTAL HEALTH ETHICS CODES

- American Association for Marriage and Family Therapy (AAMFT). (2001). *Code of Ethics* (www.aamft.org/resources/lrmplan/ethics/ethicscode2001.asp).
- American Association of Pastoral Counselors. (1994). *Code of Ethics* (www.aapc.org/ethics.cfm).
- American Counseling Association. (2005). *Code of Ethics* (www.counseling.org/Resources/CodeOfEthics/TP/Home/CT2.aspx).
- American Medical Association. (2006). Code of Medical Ethics: Current Opinions with Annotations, 2006–2007 (www.ama-assn.org/ama/pub/category/2498.html).
- American Mental Health Counselors Association. (2000). *Code of Ethics* (www.amhca.org/code).
- American Psychiatric Association. (2006). *The Principles of Medical Ethics with Annotations Especially Applicable to Psychiatry* (www.psych.org/MainMenu/PsychiatricPractice/Ethics/ResourcesStandards/PrinciplesofMedicalEthics.aspx).
- American Psychological Association. (2002). *Ethical Principles of Psychologists and Code of Conduct* (www.apa.org/ethics).
- National Association of Social Workers. (1996). *Code of Ethics* (www.socialworkers.org/pubs/codenew/code.asp).
- National Board for Certified Counselors. (2005). *Code of Ethics* (www.nbcc.org/ethics2).

Because ethics codes are designed to apply in a general manner across professional contexts, specific application of a code is often dependent upon supplementary resources, such as guidelines of professional organizations, scholarly publications, jurisdictional laws, colleagues, and ethics committees.

PROFESSIONAL GUIDELINES AND RELATED RESOURCES

Geriatric mental health professionals have many sources of moral, professional, ethical, and legal authority from which to draw when faced with ethical challenges. Ethics codes are typically written to provide clinicians with minimum acceptable standards of professional behavior and to serve as the basis for disciplinary action by professional organizations. For these reasons, clinicians tend to be aware of and generally familiar with the ethics code of their profession. However, professional organizations, and specialties within professions, often supplement their ethics codes with more specific guidelines, position statements, or policies to assist clinicians with ethical and professional decision making in specialty aspects of practice or research, such as geriatrics (see Appendix A for a list of selected guidelines). Agreement does not always exist between professional guidelines or between guidelines and ethics codes. When discrepancies between guidelines are encountered, it is typically beneficial to seek a convergence of opinions or positions from multiple sources, understanding that some resources carry more weight than others.

In addition to professional guidelines specific to geriatric mental health, resources related to more general aspects of practice that are commonly employed with older adults are valuable resources. For example, mental health professionals frequently evaluate older adults who report or present with cognitive problems. When questions arise about appropriate selection, use, and interpretation of tests, the *Standards for Educational and Psychological Testing* (American Educational Research Association, American Psychological Association, and National Council on Measurement in Education, 1999) is a primary resource. Similarly, a variety of position papers pertaining to testing-related informed consent, third-party observation, test data security, and symptom validity assessment have been provided by the National Academy of Neuropsychology (www.nanonline. org).

The settings in which mental health professionals work with older adults also provide guidelines and additional resources for determining appropriate professional conduct. For example, skilled nursing facilities typically have ethics committees and legal departments or personnel that define and enforce appropriate professional conduct. Mental health professionals who provide services in such settings should take advantage of such resources to minimize the potential for ethical misconduct, explore possibilities for pursuing ethical ideals, and better prepare themselves for addressing ethical questions or challenges when they arise. The availability of institutional ethical and legal resources can be an advantage of working in such settings.

Discrepancies between ethical requirements and guidelines regarding appropriate professional conduct occur with some frequency.

In such instances, clinicians should consider the source of each resource and weigh its relative importance accordingly. For example, an ethical requirement established by the primary professional organization of a discipline typically carries more weight than a position paper by a special interest organization. When confronted with conflicting ethical and/or professional requirements, the use of an ethical decision-making model, such as the one described in Chapter 5, often helps to clarify the preferred course of action. The ethical decision-making process includes consultation with colleagues who are experienced in addressing ethical issues, as well as reliance on multiple other ethical, legal, and professional resources.

In addition to formal guidelines, scholarly publications serve as a valuable resource for establishing and maintaining ethical practices and making ethical decisions. Books, book chapters, and articles published in journals often provide a valuable integration of philosophical reasoning, empirical evidence, and clinical experience that can assist clinicians wishing to promote their ethical competence and development.

COLLEAGUES

Experienced and informed colleagues constitute an important source of ethical information and direction. Consultation with such colleagues may occur through professional organizations or informal personal contacts. Most professional organizations have ethics committees that provide information and advice to their members. State licensing or certifying bodies are also poised to advise on ethical and legal aspects of practice and may be particularly important resources given their control over our ability to practice.

Informal consultation with colleagues who are knowledgeable about and experienced with challenging ethical issues can be a particularly strong resource. Colleagues who have served on ethics committees or written or presented on ethical matters may be well prepared to help clarify the salient ethical issues, draw upon published resources, and think through options for a good resolution to the dilemma.

In addition to collaborating with colleagues within one's profession, collaboration with colleagues across mental health disciplines can increase familiarity, comfort, and competence in the provision of patient care, which is advantageous for both patients and professionals. Interdisciplinary collaboration allows for the provision of complementary services, including the integration of areas of expertise. However, such familiarity can at times threaten ethical practice. Perhaps the greatest interdisciplinary threat to ethical practice resides in the temptation or invitation to engage in behaviors that lie beyond our limits of professional competence or scope of practice.

For example, mental health professionals without appropriate credentials to prescribe medications may nevertheless develop knowledge and familiarity with medications that are used regularly with certain patient populations and begin to feel comfortable offering advice about medication options or dosages. Similarly, clinicians who do not have the education and training to appropriately select, use, and interpret tests of mood, personality, and cognitive functioning may consider it appropriate to administer screening instruments or more extensive test batteries. In fact, some clinicians who are competent to prescribe medications or use psychometric measures may seek the assistance of less-qualified colleagues to perform needed services. However, to avoid harming patients and bringing discredit to our professions and institutions, mental health professionals must provide services only within the boundaries of our competence, based on education, training, and supervised experience. Additionally, we must not promote services by unqualified persons for the sake of expedience, convenience, or profit. Clinicians who practice under the license or supervision of another practitioner (e.g., nurse practitioners or physician's assistance) have a responsibility to seek qualified supervisors and utilize their expertise in a manner that promotes patient care. Similarly, supervisors of mental health care extenders have a responsibility to provide the amount and quality of supervision that is both consistent with applicable laws and needed by the individual care extender to ensure her competence.

Although scopes of practice describe activities in which members of a profession may engage, the professional activities of different mental health disciplines as described in their scopes of practice tend to overlap considerably, and not all members of a professional discipline are qualified to provide all of the services outlined in their scope of practice. For these reasons, it is important to consider not only the scope of practice of an individual clinician's discipline but also her competence to provide the services that she provides.

Open communication and a spirit of cooperation within and between mental health disciplines allows patients to receive an optimal combination of services and reduces the likelihood of ethical misconduct. More formal input from colleagues in the form of continuing education courses allows clinicians to learn about ethical and legal changes and the application of those changes from those who spend a considerable amount of time considering ethical matters. In some courses, the exchange of information and experiences among participants can be particularly valuable.

PROFESSIONAL LIABILITY INSURANCE CARRIERS

Professional liability (malpractice) insurance carriers typically have representatives available to consult with clinicians regarding ethical and legal matters, usually from a risk management perspective. "Risk is the calculation that a particular treatment, intervention, or service will lead to a good or bad outcome and that the outcome will have positive or negative consequences" (Bennett, Bricklin, Harris, Knapp, Vande-Creek, & Younggren, 2006, p. 11). Risk involves several factors, including patient risk characteristics, context, disciplinary consequences, and therapist factors, and there are always emotional consequences for the mental health professional involved (Bennett et al., 2006).

Three key risk management principles exist: informed consent, documentation, and consultation, each of which is linked to bioethical principles (see Bennett et al., 2006 for a review). Good risk management principles involve an integration of the ethical and legal requirements of a profession, help to promote ethical ideals, and improve the quality of patient care. Six false risk management principles also exist: (a) always get a suicidal patient to sign a safety contract; (b) try not to keep records because they can be used against you if a complaint is filed; (c) never keep detailed records when patients present a threat to harm themselves or others; (d) informed consent obligations consist only of getting the signature of patients on an informed consent form; (e) risk management is only concerned with protecting the psychologist from disciplinary actions; and (f) never self-disclose and never touch a patient (Bennett et al., 2006).

Clinicians should acknowledge that, from both clinical and risk management perspectives, (a) we will make mistakes, (b) we cannot help everyone, (c) we will not know everything, (d) we cannot go it alone, and (e) it is helpful to have a proper mix of confidence and humility (Bennett et al., 2006). The risk management principles to which we adhere should be consistent with our general orientation toward our professional activities and, like other aspects of our practice, should be congruent with our deepest personal values (Bennett et al., 2006; Pope & Vasquez, 2005). Professionals representing professional liability carriers may focus on the *4 Ds* of professional conduct that lead to licensing board complaints or malpractice suits: "the presence of a duty, the deviation from the standards of the profession, damage to the patient, and the direct connection between the deviation from duty and the damage to the patient" (Knapp & VandeCreek, 2006, p. 197).

As with all steps in the ethical decision-making process, it is important to document consultations with professional organizations and colleagues. Such documentation helps to provide structure to the decision-making process, and it can demonstrate the clinician's investment in determining an appropriate solution to an ethical dilemma in the event of an investigation by a regulatory body.

The "I Think" Problem

Geriatric mental health professionals who provide consultation to colleagues in need of ethical guidance must be aware of *The "I think" Problem*. Although there has been a significant movement toward evidence-based practice in recent years, many mental health professionals have long endorsed the scientist-practitioner model of education, training, and practice and have taken some degree of pride in making clinical decisions based on the available empirical evidence of the profession. For example, when an older adult with complaints of mild memory loss presents for the first time, the competent clinician does not simply listen to the account of the patient's problems and offer a diagnosis of a dementing disorder. Rather, the clinician will conduct a thorough interview of the patient, observe the patient, interview family members or others, perform or refer for neurodiagnostic tests, integrate the information obtained from these various sources, consider all diagnostic possibilities, review relevant literature and consult with colleagues as needed, and then offer a diagnostic impression.

In contrast, when it comes to an ethical decision, I frequently hear those same colleagues begin their responses to complex ethical questions with the words "I think." For example, "I think you should . . . ." It is rare to have a colleague reply to a complex ethical question with a statement along the lines of the following: "Based on ethical standard X, state law Y, position paper Z, my clinical experience, and my knowledge of how you feel about such issues, an appropriate course of action would be . . . ." As with the movement toward empirically based therapeutic decision making, we need to adopt an empirically based approach to ethical decision making.

EVIDENCE-BASED BIOETHICS AND THE EVOLUTION OF PROFESSIONAL ETHICS

Like other aspects of clinical practice and research, the establishment of ethically appropriate behavior is an evolutionary process. Ethics codes are updated periodically, with old standards being preserved, updated, or eliminated, and new standards added. The dynamic nature of professional ethics codes and guidelines results from multiple factors, including gradual changes in shared values, professional-political influences, legal matters, changes in professional activities due to technological advances, and the biases of the individuals or groups in positions of influence.

As described in the preceding section, ethical analysis and decision making have long been guided by philosophical principles, theological positions, normative morality, and subjective assumptions. Although such a theoretical approach to professional ethics has considerable value as a foundation for professional behavior, and must be relied upon to guide specific behaviors in the absence of empirical evidence, recent research has demonstrated that some long-held assumptions are unfounded, and this has tipped the scales of controversy for long-debated topics. Seemingly logical clinical insights may end up being seriously flawed when subjected to scientific scrutiny (Halpern, 2005).

EVIDENCE-BASED ETHICS

The results of empirical studies, although not without their potential limitations, add an element of objectivity to what may otherwise be a very subjective philosophical endeavor. For example, neuropsychology as a specialty has long been of the opinion that having third parties (e.g., family members, supervisors, attorneys, roommates, recording devices) present during neurocognitive testing affects the patient's performance and is therefore not appropriate. However, until relatively recently, this position was based on the subjective opinions of clinicians and was thus the subject of some controversy. With the publication of a series of studies by Robert McCaffrey and his colleagues, as well as other investigators (Constantinou, Ashendorf, & McCaffrey, 2002; Constantinou, Ashendorf, & McCaffrey, 2005; Gavett, Lynch, & McCaffrey, 2005; Kehrer, Sanchez, Habif, Rosenbaum, & Townes, 2000; McCaffrey, 2005; Lynch, 2005; McCaffrey, Lynch, & Yantz, 2005; Yantz & McCaffrey, 2006), a body of empirical evidence now documents the significant adverse impact that third-party observers have on neurocognitive test performance. Although the nature and appropriateness of third-party observers in some neuropsychological evaluation contexts remains a matter of some debate (Blase, 2008), the emergence of a body of empirical evidence that addresses this question has advanced the discussion and understanding of this topic significantly.

Halpern (2005) described, as examples of the value of basing ethical decisions on empirical evidence, studies of the impact of financial enticements on decisions to become research participants. It has been argued that paying individuals to be research subjects represents an undue inducement, because when confronted with money, some people will not fully consider the risks of participation, resulting in consent to participate that is not fully informed and not consistent with the principle of autonomy (Dickert & Grady, 1999; Grady, 2001; Macklin, 1981; McGee, 1997; McNeil, 1997; Viens, 2001; Wilkenson & Moore, 1997). However, preliminary empirical investigations of this issue revealed that participants' determinations of the importance of risk were not lessened when offered more money (Halpern, Karlawish, Casarett, Berlin, & Asch, 2004). Rather, the risk of being a research subject was consistent across different levels of payment (Bentley & Thacker, 2004; Halpern et al., 2004). Additionally, contrary to expectation (Viens, 2001), lower-income participants were influenced less by payment amount than were participants with higher socioeconomic status (Halpern et al., 2004). Thus, these empirical investigations shed doubt on long-held beliefs about problems with paying research subjects.

Continued and expanded empirical study of ethical issues is needed to reduce reliance on subjective resources. Ethics resources that are based on perception, experience, or opinion may be unintentionally swayed in a direction that is later found to lack empirical support or may be intentionally influenced by groups or individuals with personal agendas that may not be consistent with the best interests of patients, society, or the mental health professions. For topics that are amenable to empirical investigation, "position papers" of professional organizations that rely on as yet unverified opinions should be considered hypothesis-generating until the issues have been appropriately investigated (Halpern, 2005).

Empirically based ethics, although appealing for the reasons just described, are not without controversy, as evidenced by reactions to Halpern's (2005) article (see www.bmj.com/cgi/eletters/331/7521/901). What seems to be beyond dispute, to the extent that anything in ethics can be, is that both philosophical and empirical approaches to ethical decision making serve important roles and, when possible, should be considered together to produce balanced, informed professional choices.

As with clinical decision making, ethical decision making should be based on empirical evidence to the extent that such evidence exists. Such evidence may be particularly important when establishing ethics policies (Kim, 2004). Additional funding may help generate research into ethical issues that have previously been considered beyond the realm of empirical investigation.

POSITIVE ETHICS

Ethical and legal *requirements* establish a minimum level of professional responsibility. Remedial ethics focus on enforcing these minimum requirements; that is, failure to meet these requirements serves as the basis for disciplinary action. In contrast, ethical *principles* and professional *guidelines* are generally considered *aspirational*, reflecting a higher level of professional responsibility and thus a higher degree of protection of the rights of patients and their families and the public. Although enforceable requirements can be distinguished from aspirational guidelines, it is difficult to conceive of clinical situations in which geriatric mental health professionals would be justified in simply pursuing a minimum level of ethical conduct. Geriatric mental health practitioners should aspire and strive to achieve and maintain a level of professional conduct that reflects the highest standards of ethical practice.

Positive ethics represents shift in emphasis from misconduct and disciplinary action to the active promotion of exemplary behavior (Handelsman, Knapp, & Gottlieb, 2002; Knapp & VandeCreek, 2004, 2006). Positive ethics requires clinicians to examine the perspectives and process that allow maximum adherence to moral principles (Knapp & VandeCreeek, 2006). However, such examination of oneself, one's professional behavior, and the wide array of behavioral and philosophical options can be a time- and labor-intensive process.

Some clinicians choose not to pursue ethical ideals because maintaining a high standard of ethical conduct requires time and expense beyond that required by minimum enforceable standards. For example, in New York State, mental health professionals are not required to participate in continuing education (www.op.nysed.gov/part29.htm#mhp); that is, they are on the honor system with regard to maintaining professional competence. As a result, clinicians vary widely in the degree to which they remain informed about advances in the knowledge, skills, and procedures that are the foundation of clinical practice.

Although clinicians who choose the least extensive professional development options may maintain a minimum level of competence, they and their patients will likely derive less benefit than will clinicians who are members of professional organizations, receive and read journals, attend conferences, and engage in other forms of structured continuing education on a consistent basis. Thus, although there are mandates for mental health professionals in New York State to maintain competence in professional activities, the decision of whether to participate in continuing education resides with the clinician. "The pursuit of ethical ideals requires an allocation of time and effort that only a personal commitment to such ideals can support . . . a personal commitment to ethical ideals is a primary responsibility and obligation of all practitioners" (Bush & Martin, 2006; p. 64). Geriatric mental health professionals in New York State who are committed to pursuing ethical ideals will actively and regularly seek both formal and informal avenues of continuing education.

Trends by hospital staff credentialing committees and board certification specialty boards (added qualifications) toward increased emphasis on maintaining professional competence help to ensure that clinicians continue their professional development, which is particularly valuable in jurisdictions that do not require documentation of formal continuing education. Ultimately, each clinician must decide for herself the extent to which high standards of ethical practice are important and the amount of personal resources (time, effort, money) that are worth investing in ethical practice.

Learning Exercises

1. List in order the top five resources that you would consult when anticipating or confronting an ethical dilemma. Is the order flexible? Why or why not? Use examples to illustrate your position.

2. Describe the relationship between societal values, general bioethical principles, and professional ethics codes.

3 Legal Issues

Ethical practice and legal practice are not synonymous (Bricklin, 2001). The clinical practices of mental health professionals are governed by state and Federal laws. Although violations of the ethical standards of professional organizations can result in censure by, or expulsion from, the organization, violations of law can result in the loss of one's license to practice and criminal prosecution. Nevertheless, many mental health practitioners are more familiar with their professional ethics codes than they are with the laws governing their professional behavior. Fortunately for such practitioners, ethics codes often are more conservative than laws, providing protections for consumers and the public that extend beyond the legal requirements. As a result, practitioners who comply with their professional ethics code are also likely to comply with laws; however, exceptions to this general rule exist, requiring knowledge of both ethics and law.

JURISDICTIONAL CONSIDERATIONS

Individual licensing or certification bodies may adopt, in whole or in part, the ethics code of a given discipline for that discipline's legally mandated rules of professional conduct. This practice reduces the potential for conflict between ethical and legal requirements. For example, in psychology, some states have adopted the American Psychological Association's (2002a) *Ethical Principles of Psychologists and Code of Conduct*, some states have adopted the Association of State and Provincial Psychology Boards' (2005) *Code of Conduct*, and others states have developed their own rules for professional conduct. Clinicians must be familiar with the laws governing their professional conduct.

FEDERAL LEGISLATION AND LITIGATION

In addition to state laws, Federal laws also protect the rights of older recipients of mental health services. The Older Americans Act (OAA), originally passed in 1965 and most recently amended in 2006 (U.S. Department of Health and Human Services, Administration on Aging, 2006), reinforces the American value of dignity as an inherent right of older adults, establishes entitlements to which older adults must have an equal opportunity for full and free enjoyment, and tasks the U.S. government with duties and responsibilities to promote the dignity of older Americans. The entitlements covered by the OAA include adequate income in retirement; access to the best possible physical and mental health services; suitable housing; restorative care in institutions and maintenance services in the home, including family and caregiver support; employment without discrimination based on age; retirement in health, honor, and dignity; opportunities to participate in, or contribute to, a wide range of meaningful activities; immediate benefits of proven research knowledge that can sustain and improve health and happiness; autonomy in planning and managing their own lives; and protection from abuse, neglect, and exploitation (42 U.S.C. 3001).

Mental health professionals routinely work with older adults, their loved ones, and others to promote the dignity of the older adult in the ways addressed by the OAA. Clinical and ethical decision making should include consideration of these freedoms and securities to which older adult patients are entitled. It is in this context that elder abuse reporting laws and procedures are encountered. All geriatric mental health professionals should be familiar with the elder abuse reporting laws and procedures for their jurisdiction (see www.aarp.org/bulletin/yourlife/statebystate_elder_abuse_resource_list. html for a list of elder abuse resources for each state).

Because aging is associated with increased medical problems that significantly affect emotional state, the Americans with Disabilities Act (ADA, 1990) may be particularly relevant for mental health professionals in a variety of medical and mental health treatment contexts. The ADA was created to provide legislative support for the prevention of discrimination against people with disabilities and for the promotion of participation in society by individuals with disabilities. The ADA addresses five areas: employment, public services, public accommodations, transportation, and telecommunications. Although the ADA originally was considered to be landmark civil rights legislation, the ADA has been interpreted somewhat narrowly by the U.S. Supreme Court (Gostin, 2003). Mental health professionals, particularly those in medical and rehabilitative settings, "need to have a thorough understanding of the Americans with Disabilities Act to be effective advocates for their patients' vocational reentry and to meet their professional responsibilities under the principles of beneficence and justice" (Hanson, Kerkhoff, & Bush, 2005; p. 179).

Additionally, the Health Insurance Portability and Accountability Act of 1996 (HIPAA; U.S. Department of Health and Human Services, 2003) grants patients certain rights to privacy and to review and amend their records. Clinicians should consult their state laws and institutional resources and determine HIPAA's applicability to their practices. A variety of resources (e.g., Zur, 2005) exist to help the private practitioner understand and comply with HIPAA requirements.

Federal legislation for financial matters, such as the Omnibus Budget Reconciliation Acts (OBRAs) of 1987 and 1989 and the Balanced Budget Act (BBA) of 1997 (P.L. 105-33), has had direct effects on the provision and reception of mental health services. The OBRAs addressed some of the problems with Medicare, such as raising reimbursement and eliminating the cap on the number of outpatient mental health sessions allowed. The BBA established Medicare Part C (Medicare Plus Choice) as managed care option for those eligible for Medicare, but the program was never widely accepted, and the number of enrollees has declined over the years. Although these acts addressed some concerns of older adults with mental health needs, problems, confusion, and disagreement regarding some aspects remain (see Reichman, Streim, & Loebel, 2004, for a review).

For more than a decade, mental health care providers and organizations have worked to end the discriminatory health insurance coverage that provides greater benefits for medical care than mental health care. The goal of parity legislation is to close the gap between physical and mental health care insurance benefits. Congress passed the Mental Health Parity Act (P.L. 104-204) in 1996, which mandated that companies with more than 50 employees provide equivalent annual and lifetime insurance coverage amounts for mental health care and medical care. However, many employers and insurers violated the spirit of the law by utilizing loopholes in the law that allow them to place other restrictions on mental health benefits. Such restrictions include limiting the number of covered outpatient office visits and number of days for inpatient care, and limiting the diagnoses that are covered. In the past decade, repeated legislative efforts in Congress to close the loopholes have generated widespread bipartisan support. Additionally, state-level parity laws have been adopted in many states to address restrictions on mental health care coverage that are not addressed in the federal Mental Health Parity Act, although the scope of the laws varies from state to state (www.aarp.org/research/health/carequality/aresearch-import-676-FS69.html).

On March 5, 2007, the U.S. House of Representatives passed the Paul Wellstone Mental Health and Addiction Equity Act of 2007 (HR 1424) (http://thomas.loc.gov/cgi-bin/query/z?c110:H.R.1424:). Then, on September 18, 2007, the Senate unanimously passed the Mental Health Parity Act of 2007 (S. 558) (http://thomas.loc.gov/cgi-bin/query/z?c110:S.558:). Although there are differences in the House and Senate bills, they are similar in that they both preserve strong parity and consumer protection laws at the state level while extending federal parity protections. These bills bring the United States closer to establishing treatment benefits for millions of individuals with mental health and substance use disorders that are equal to medical benefits. The Congressional Budget Office projects that

House and Senate parity bills would raise average health plan costs by only 0.4%, which would be shared by the employer and employee, with the employer typically paying a third of the total. At present, a strong push is under way by the mental health community to encourage Congress to pass these bills into law (e.g., www.apapractice.org/apo/in_the_news/house_passes_parity.html#).

The Centers for Medicare and Medicaid Services (CMS; previously the Health Care Financing Administration [HCFA]) hold the purse strings for medical and mental health services for many older adults and the clinicians and institutions that provide services. As such, they wield considerable influence with regard to the regulation of mental health services, providing mandates for certain types of coverage and quality indicators, and the documentation that goes with it. For example, a clear Federal mandate exists for the detection and treatment of mental illness in residents of nursing homes (HCFA, 1992; Reichman et al., 2004), although such a mandate does not mean that competent psychiatric services will be available (Colenda, Bartels, & Gottlieb, 1999; Reichman et al., 1998). Federal funding through the Department of Veterans Affairs also supports mental health care for a large number of older adults. Clinicians working within such facilities or systems must be familiar with the regulations that govern such practice.

Skilled nursing facilities became a ready alternative to psychiatric hospitals for older adults with serious mental illness during the movement to deinstitutionalize psychiatric inpatients. Because of the inappropriateness of nursing homes for such patients (OBRA-87; U.S. Department of Health and Human Services, Office of the Inspector General, 2001), increased efforts have been made in recent years to increase options for older adults with serious mental illness to remain in their homes or in other community settings (*Olmstead v. L.C.*, 1999; Williams, 2000).

Individuals have the right to express their wishes regarding life-sustaining care, such as artificial hydration and nutrition, and to have those wishes respected (*Cruzan v. Director*, 1990; Patient Self-Determination Act, 1991; *Washington v. Glucksberg*, 1997). Hospitals, skilled nursing facilities, and other facilities that receive Medicare and Medicaid funds must, upon admission, notify patients of their right to express their wishes, including their rights as granted by the state to establish advance directives. For those patients who have had artificial life-sustaining treatment initiated, they or their proxy have the legal right to discontinue such treatment with the knowledge that it will result in the patient's death. Courts have rejected the distinction between withholding and withdrawing life-sustaining treatments (*Barber v. Superior Court*, 1983; *Brophy v. New England Sinai Hospital Inc.*, 1986). The discontinuation of feeding at the request of the patient or proxy has not been determined to be suicide or active euthanasia but rather to be allowing the underlying medical condition to run its natural course (Reichman et al., 2004). These cases clearly reflect the primary value that the courts place on self-determination and the importance of respecting autonomy in the context of terminal illness.

CONFLICTS BETWEEN ETHICAL AND LEGAL RESOURCES

The ethical and legal requirements that govern the professional conduct of geriatric mental health practitioners are generally congruent. However, in some circumstances, discrepancies between the various authoritative resources exist, particularly given the differences among state laws regarding professional conduct. As a result, clinicians should not rely solely on their familiarity with one resource, such as the code of ethics of their discipline.

Geriatric mental health professionals must have an understanding of both the ethics and laws that govern their practice. For example, the neuropsychological examination of older adults with disabilities at times requires deviations from standardized test administration (e.g., providing visual presentation of a word list for patients who are extremely hard of hearing) be made in order for the construct of interest (e.g., memory) to be adequately examined. When the reliability and validity of tests administered with such accommodations have not been established, the American Psychological Association's (2002a) Ethics Code requires clinicians to describe the strengths and limitations of test results and interpretation and to identify any significant limitations on their interpretations (Ethical Standards 9.02, Use of Assessments, and 9.06, Interpreting Assessment Results). Such description of limitations requires the examiner to identify or "flag" the patient's disability. However, the Rehabilitation Act of 1973 prohibits the flagging of accommodations; that is, the clinician must not identify the use of, or reason for, testing accommodations, apparently to help protect the patient from discrimination that may occur if identified as disabled. When faced with conflicting requirements such as this, it can be helpful to turn to other relevant resources.

The Standards for Educational and Psychological Testing (SEPT) (Standard 10.11) provide additional information for the clinician struggling with how to handle this situation. According to the SEPT, in the absence of established comparability between test scores obtained with and without an accommodation, "specific information about the nature of the modification should be provided, if permitted by law, to assist test users to properly interpret and act on test scores." However, the Comment section that follows Standard 10.11 states that the report should contain no reference to the existence or nature of the test taker's disability. In their chapter on this challenging subject, Caplan and Shechter (2005) stated, "As worded, this standard seems to us to be a 'Catch 22,' imposing a considerable burden on the psychologist to describe and justify the modification that directly stemmed from the disability without naming the disability" (p. 100).

With the goal of protecting and promoting patient and public welfare, the first obligation for geriatric mental health professionals is to meet both ethical and legal requirements. However, when conflicts between ethical and legal requirements are encountered, clinicians should make known their commitment to professional ethics and attempt to resolve the matter in a manner consistent with their ethics code. If an ethically preferable solution or compromise cannot be reached, clinicians should ultimately yield to the legal authority. When conflicts between different legal requirements are encountered, clinicians should consider which law offers the greatest protection of safety or other relevant rights and *consult legal counsel* as needed. The promotion of ethical and legal conduct is maximized by considering bioethical principles and ethical and legal resources in the context of a personal commitment to the pursuit of ethical ideals.

Pope, Tabachnick, and Keith-Spiegel (1987) and Gibson and Pope (1993) surveyed psychologists and national certified counselors, respectively, regarding ethical beliefs and behaviors, as well as the value they placed in various resources for ethical decision making. When engaged in ethical decision making, the mental health professionals surveyed listed their professional ethics code and the perspectives of colleagues among their most highly valued resources, whereas laws, scholarly ethics publications, and local ethics committees were among those resources valued least (see Table 3.1 for complete ratings).

To help coordinate ethical requirements with other practice guidelines for psychologists and psychiatrists invested in maintaining responsible professional behavior, Redlich and Pope (1980) offered the following seven principles: (1) above all, do no harm; (2) practice only with competence; (3) do not exploit; (4) treat people with respect for their dignity as human beings; (5) protect confidentiality; (6) act, except in the most extreme instances, only after obtaining informed consent; and (7) practice, insofar as possible, within the framework of social equity and justice. The first five principles have their roots in ancient medicine and are reflected in the Hippocratic Oath, whereas

Table 3.1

VALUE RATINGS FOR ETHICAL RESOURCES[a]

HIGHEST RATED/MOST HELPFUL	LOWEST RATED/LEAST HELPFUL
Colleagues	Local ethics committees
Ethics Codes (APA, AACD/ACA[b])	Published clinical/theoretical work/research
Internship training	State and Federal laws
AACD/ACA Ethics Committee	Court decisions
Journal of Counseling & Development	Agencies for which participants had worked
State licensing boards	

[a]Combined results from Pope et al. (1987) and Gibson & Pope, 1993. The order in which the resources are presented does not imply order of importance.
[b]The AACD (American Association for Counseling and Development) became the ACA (American Counseling Association)
APA, American Psychological Association

the sixth and seventh principles originated more recently, focus more on patients' rights, and have not, according to Redlich and Pope at the time of their publication, achieved acceptance equal to the first five principles. Keeping these principles in mind will help mental health professionals to anticipate, avoid, and more successfully address ethical dilemmas.

Learning Exercises

1. The Older Americans Act does all of the following, except:

   a. reinforce the American value of dignity as an inherent right of older adults.
   b. establish entitlements to which older adults must have an equal opportunity for full and free enjoyment.
   c. task the U.S. government with duties and responsibilities to promote the dignity of older Americans.
   d. mandate that by the year 2015 all U.S. sidewalks have curb cuts so that they are wheelchair accessible.

2. Which of the following contexts became a ready alternative to psychiatric hospitals for older adults with serious mental illness during the movement in the United States to deinstitutionalize psychiatric inpatients?

   a. The Army
   b. Assisted living facilities
   c. Skilled nursing facilities
   d. None of the above; most older adults with serious mental illness were left homeless

3. True/False. When surveyed by Pope, Tabachnick, and Keith-Spiegel (1987) and Gibson and Pope (1993), mental health professionals reported that when they are engaged in ethical decision making, they prefer to turn first to their jurisdictional laws (so that they stay out of jail), then their liability insurance carrier (so that they don't get sued), followed by their professional ethics code and colleagues.

4   Salient Ethical Issues

The ethical concerns of geriatric mental health professionals vary across clinical settings and patient populations. Although the ethical concerns of clinicians who work with older adults overlap with the concerns of those who work with younger populations, there can be different emphases and unique considerations. To understand the salient ethical issues in context, it is helpful to first review the ethical concerns and dilemmas encountered by members of mental health professions more generally. Familiarity with the salient ethical issues in mental health practice generally and in geriatric mental health specifically allows us to anticipate ethically troubling situations, informs our decision making, and guides our education and training.

To investigate the types of ethical dilemmas encountered in the day-to-day work of psychologists, Pope and Vetter (1992) surveyed 1,319 members of the American Psychological Association and requested examples of ethical dilemmas that the psychologists encountered in their work. The dilemmas were grouped into 23 general categories representing the ethical and practice areas of concern. The top five categories of concern for psychologists were confidentiality; blurred, dual, or conflictual relationships; payment sources, plans, settings, and methods; academic, teaching, and training issues; and forensic issues. Concerns related to assessment ranked ninth, and professional competence ranked eleventh.

Because of the considerable involvement of neuropsychologists in answering diagnostic questions that commonly emerge in late adulthood and providing recommendations or follow-up services, the experiences and concerns of this specialty area of practice regarding ethical issues are of particular relevance to geriatric mental health practice. The ethical concerns of psychologists specializing in neuropsychology diverge from concerns of the general membership of the American Psychological Association. In a review of ethically challenging vignettes elicited from members of the American Board of Clinical Neuropsychology, the greatest percentage (56%) of ethical problems involved aspects of assessment practices (Brittain, Francis, & Barth, 1995). From a more theoretical and experiential perspective, Bush (2007) described 12 common sources of ethical conflict in clinical neuropsychology. Table 4.1 compares the top 12 areas of ethical concern for psychologists in general (Pope & Vetter, 1992) with those most relevant to neuropsychology (Bush, 2007; Bush, Grote, Johnson-Greene, & Macartney-Filgate, 2008). Table 4.1 not only provides common sources of ethical concern but also illustrates those differences in the issues that are considered most challenging by clinicians in different types of clinical activities and with different patient populations.

With regard to ethical issues in *geriatric* neuropsychology specifically, issues that have been emphasized include the need for professional competence, the unique assessment considerations, and the importance of respect for people's rights and dignity, all aimed at the promotion of the client's welfare (Bush & Martin, 2005; McSweeny, 2005; Morgan, 2002, 2005). Additional publications have reviewed ethical issues in neuropsychology in practice settings in which elderly patients are frequently encountered, such as acute medical settings (Pinkston, 2005; Wilde, 2005; Wilde, Bush, & Zeifert, 2002) and rehabilitation settings (DeLuca, 2005; Johnson-Greene, 2005; Swiercinsky, 2002).

Pope, Tabachnick, and Keith-Spiegel (1987) and Gibson and Pope (1993) took a more behavior-focused approach in their investigations

Table 4.1

COMMON SOURCES OF ETHICAL CONCERN FOR PSYCHOLOGISTS AND NEUROPSYCHOLOGISTS

PSYCHOLOGISTS[a]	NEUROPSYCHOLOGISTS[b]
1. Confidentiality	Professional competence
2. Blurred, dual, or conflictual relationships	Roles/relationships (dual/multiple)
3. Payment sources, plans, settings, and methods	Test security/release of raw test data
4. Academic settings, teaching dilemmas, and concerns about training	Third-party observers
5. Forensic psychology	Confidentiality
6. Research	Assessment
7. Conduct of colleagues	Conflicts between ethics and law
8. Sexual issues	False or deceptive statements
9. Assessment	Objectivity
10. Questionable or harmful interventions	Cooperation with other professionals
11. Competence	Informed consent/third-party requests for services
12. Ethics (and related) codes and committees	Record keeping and fees

[a]From Ethical dilemmas encountered by members of the American Psychologic Association: A national survey, by K. S., Pope, & V. A., Vetter, 1992, *American Psychologist, 47,* 397–411, with permission. Table 1: Categories of 703 Ethically Troubling Incidents. The top 12 of Pope's and Vetter's total of 23 general categories are listed here. The categories are based on survey data from 679 psychologists.
[b]From *Ethical Decision Making in Clinical Neuropsychology,* by S. S., Bush, 2007, New York: Oxford University Press, with permission. The categories are based on the combination of interviews of ethically knowledgeable neuropsychologists (Bush et al., in press b), review of the literature, and the author's clinical experiences.

of ethical concerns. Pope and colleagues (1987) collected data regarding the degree to which psychologists engaged in each of 83 behaviors and the degree to which they considered each behavior to be ethical. Similarly, Gibson and Pope surveyed a national sample of 1,000 counselors certified by the National Board for Certified Counselors. They achieved a 59.7% return rate from counselors indicating their beliefs about whether each of 88 behaviors was ethical and the degree to which they were confident of their judgment about the behavior. Although a review of the specific findings of these studies is beyond the scope of this chapter, readers are encouraged to review the comprehensive normative data that they provide regarding the behaviors of mental health professionals and the relationships of the behaviors to ethical standards. Such data help inform clinicians when making choices about their own behavior and the actions of colleagues.

Although ethical concerns, challenges, and opportunities may emerge in any aspect of clinical practice or research with older adults, just as they may with younger patient populations, certain themes and variations are encountered more when working with older adults. Consistent themes in the writings about ethics in geriatric medicine and mental health include autonomy, cognitive capacity, and informed consent; privacy and confidentiality; relationships and conflicts of interest with others and institutions; advocacy; accommodations and special precautions; and professional clinical and ethical competence (Ables, 2006; American Psychological Association, 2004; Blank 2004; Eliopoulos, 1987; Feinsod & Wagner, 2007; Fitting, 1986; Holstein & McCurdy, 1999; Knight, 2004; Lichtenberg et al., 1998; Rai, 1999; Sachs & Cassel, 1994; Wicclair, 1993).

In this volume, eight aspects of geriatric mental health practice that seem likely to generate considerable opportunity for the examination of ethical issues are presented (see Table 4.2). Section II centers around these eight aspects of practice. Although these aspects of practice may seem applicable to nearly all mental health specialties, and

Table 4.2

ASPECTS OF GERIATRIC MENTAL HEALTH PRACTICE THAT REQUIRE CONSIDERABLE ETHICAL ATTENTION

1. Professional Competence
2. Human Relations
3. Privacy, Confidentiality, and Informed Consent
4. Assessment
5. Treatment
6. Serving Special Populations
7. Health Promotion
8. Social Considerations

some may appear to be rather general, it is through the application of these aspects of mental health practice to our work with older adults that their unique contributions and ethical importance emerge.

Learning Exercises

1. True/False. Compared to neuropsychologists, psychologists generally are more concerned about ethical challenges stemming from confidentiality than from professional competence.

2. List the top five threats to ethical practice that you are most likely to encounter in your practice.

3. List the top five threats to ethical practice that you are most likely to observe in the practices of your geriatric mental health colleagues.

5 | Ethical Decision Making

When considering ethical issues, it would be nice if there were "bottom-line" answers to ethical questions and problems. Of course, the answers to some ethical questions, such as whether a mental health professional should have sex with a patient, are so obvious that a good decision can be made quickly and easily (i.e., Don't do it!). The answers to such questions regarding whether the behaviors are appropriate typically do not pose dilemmas for clinicians. However, neither laws, ethics codes, nor position papers can answer every question that geriatric mental health professionals may encounter. Compared to relatively straightforward ethical requirements, ethical dilemmas require more analysis and are thus more time- and energy-consuming. As a result, clinicians must have a method for considering and weighing various resources to achieve good solutions. Ethical decision making at its best is typically more a process than an event.

ETHICAL DECISION-MAKING GOALS

Professional ethics are established for the protection and promotion of the well-being of others, ourselves, our professions, and society.

Consistent with the pursuit of those goals, clinicians typically engage in ethical decision making for four reasons: to anticipate and prepare for ethical issues commonly encountered in our specific practice contexts, to avoid ethical misconduct, to address ethical challenges when they are encountered, and to aspire to higher standards of ethical practice. Thus, these four general reasons for engaging in ethical decision making, which I refer to as the *4 A's* of ethical practice and decision making, are *Anticipate, Avoid, Address*, and *Aspire*. Frequent review of, and commitment to, the 4 A's of ethical practice and decision making promotes sound ethical practice.

Keeping in mind that sound ethical practice goes hand-in-hand with sound clinical practice can help geriatric mental health professionals to help others. A structured, resource-based ethical decision-making process advances clinicians in their pursuit of their ethical decision-making goals. The ability to make sound ethical decisions through a structured and informed decision-making process is facilitated through the use of an ethical decision-making model.

DECISION-MAKING MODELS

Making good decisions and determining optimal courses of action in the context of ethical uncertainty can be difficult, particularly when the ethical principles to which we turn for guidance conflict with each other. When confronting such dilemmas, use of an ethical decision-making model can be particularly valuable. A number of models have been proposed to facilitate the decision-making process when questions emerge regarding the ethical appropriateness of one's own activities or the activities of colleagues (e.g., Bush, Connell, & Denney, 2006; Deiden & Bush, 2002; Haas & Malouf, 2002; Kitchener, 2000; Knapp & Vandecreek, 2003; Koocher & Keith-Spiegel, 1998).

The model presented here is adapted from Bush, Connell, and Denney (2006) to be more specific to geriatric mental health. Specifically, new steps 3 and 4 have been inserted to take into account the unique patient and family/caregiver characteristics that can be so important with older adults, as well as the importance of determining to whom obligations are owed, whether they are the patient, a health care proxy, an institution, and/or society. These considerations seem to have greater relevance with geriatric populations than with younger adult mental health patients. Consisting of 10 steps (see Table 5.1), the proposed model is more comprehensive and detailed than most of the other models referenced. The application of this model may aid clinicians in avoiding ethical misconduct and pursuing ethical ideals.

Table 5.1

ETHICAL DECISION-MAKING STEPS

1. Identify the problem.
2. Consider the significance of the context and setting.
3. Determine patient and family/caregiver assets and limitations.
4. Consider obligations owed.
5. Identify and utilize ethical and legal resources.
6. Consider personal beliefs and values.
7. Develop possible solutions to the problem.
8. Consider the potential consequences of various solutions.
9. Choose and implement a course of action.
10. Assess the outcome and implement changes as needed.

DOCUMENTATION

The importance of documenting the efforts made and the steps taken throughout the ethical decision-making process cannot be over-stated. Documentation can help structure the clinician's approach to the decision-making process, clarify options, facilitate reasoning, and avoid omissions or redundant efforts. In addition, documentation of one's ethical decision-making efforts and commitment to ethical practice is critical if one's actions are later reviewed by an adjudicating body.

The outline of the ethical decision-making model provides a ready framework for documentation that can be supplemented with the details of the specific situation, including descriptions of the resources consulted and the reasoning underlying one's choice of action. In addition to promoting and demonstrating ethical conduct in a given situation, documentation of one's ethical decision-making process can facilitate future problem-solving in similar cases and serve as a valuable resource for colleagues facing similar challenges, as well as learning opportunities for students or trainees entering the field.

Case 1

Brian, a social worker recently hired by a skilled nursing facility, is tasked with conducting intake interviews of all residents to determine their social history, emotional adjustment, and cognitive status. Interviews with family members and the administration of emotional and cognitive screening tests are typically part of the process. When indicated, Brian provides psychotherapy for residents and their families.

Brian enters the room of Mr. A on the day of Mr. A's admission to the facility. Brian greets Mr. A's roommate and the roommate's wife on his way to Mr. A's bed. Mr. A is awake, talking to his wife and adult son and glancing at a ball game on his roommate's TV. Brian introduces himself to Mrs. A, the son, and Mr. A. He then asks Mrs. A about her husband's social history, which includes only a 6th grade education, and current problems and adjustment. He is about to administer the Mini-Mental State Exam (MMSE) and the Geriatric Depression Scale (GDS) when he considers that maybe testing should be postponed because of the distractions in the room, including the presence of other people. However, the necessity of completing intake evaluations, including obtaining the test results, on the day of admission was emphasized to him when he was hired, and he feels pressured to complete his intake while he has the chance. Unsure what to do, he excuses himself and returns to his office in search of answers.

IDENTIFY THE PROBLEM(S)

One of the primary hurdles for Brian involves issues of privacy and confidentiality. Mr. A's family is present, which can be very helpful with Brian's pursuit of background information. However, the quality of the relationships is unknown at this time, and Mr. A may not be completely open and honest with his wife and son in the room. When considering these issues, Brian realizes that he had turned to Mrs. A for information about Mr. A, rather than speaking to Mr. A directly, a choice that could have significant adverse repercussions for his relationship with Mr. A. Additionally, Mr. A's roommate and his roommate's wife are in the room, which may also make Mr. A hesitant about expressing his thoughts and feelings.

A second problem involves the selection and appropriate use of psychological and cognitive tests. Brian wonders whether he can obtain valid test results given the distractions in the room. Brain is relatively new to his job and does not know how to handle the situation; however, he knows enough to know that he needs consultation.

CONSIDER THE SIGNIFICANCE OF THE CONTEXT AND SETTING

One of Brian's most important responsibilities is to gather important information about new residents such as Mr. A as quickly as possible after admission to the facility. Such information facilitates decisions that he and other staff members must make to promote Mr. A's care and treatment. Brian knows that he may have a brief window of time in which to gather the information, because the medical and nursing staff, therapists, dietician, and others will also need to meet with Mr. A, and, like many new residents, Mr. A may fatigue quickly and need to sleep before long. Thus, there is some urgency to completing the intake evaluation.

Mr. A has a roommate who is in bed and cannot easily be transferred to a wheelchair and removed from the room. Additionally, Mr. A cannot be taken out of the room at this time. Therefore, in this setting, intake interviews and testing must often be completed with a new resident's roommate present. Also, because other staff members will need to meet with Mr. A, there may be interruptions during Brian's intake interview and testing.

DETERMINE PATIENT AND FAMILY/CAREGIVER ASSETS AND LIMITATIONS

Mr. A is alert, so Brian does not need to rush the evaluation in order to complete it before Mr. A needs to sleep. Also, Mr. A appears to have adequate hearing, so Brian does not have to speak particularly loudly, and Mr. A does not respond in an exceptionally loud voice. However, Mr. A seems to be easily distracted by his roommate's television.

Mr. A's wife and son seem to be friendly, caring, and supportive, and they seem to want to be closely involved in Mr. A's care. Such involvement can be very helpful, but it can also prove challenging when there is a need to meet and exchange information with Mr. A individually.

CONSIDER OBLIGATIONS OWED

Brian has obligations to (1) Mr. A; (2) the other staff members who depend on the psychosocial history and test results; and (3) the facility, which has requirements that must be met to maintain accreditation. Brian will also likely have an obligation to work and exchange information with Mr. A's family.

IDENTIFY AND UTILIZE ETHICAL AND LEGAL RESOURCES

Brian begins by consulting with his supervisor. Rather than simply telling him what to do, she takes an educational approach and provides him with valuable published resources, which she has accumulated over the years.

Brian first considers the *Code of Ethics* of the National Association of Social Workers (NASW, 1999). He notes in Ethical Standard (ES) 1.01 (Commitment to Clients) that his primary responsibility is to promote the welfare of the residents. He also notes in the Code that he should respect Mr. A's right to privacy and discuss any foreseeable limits to confidentiality (ES 1.07, Privacy and Confidentiality), so that Mr. A can make an informed decision about the information that he will share or withhold (ES 1.03, Informed Consent). Brian is already well aware that confidential communications involving social workers are covered under both regulatory and statutory law (Wulach, 1993). By reviewing the ethics code, Brian is also reminded that he has a responsibility to adhere to the commitments that he made to the facility when he was hired (ES 3.09, Commitments to Employers). Brian reviews the section on Evaluation and Research (ES 5.02), but does not find information specific to testing cognition or mood.

Brian next turns to the *Standards for Psychological Services in Long-Term Care Facilities* (Lichtenberg et al., 1998). In Standard V (Ethical Issues), section C (Privacy), he finds the following information:

> When no consulting room is available or the patient is bedridden, services may be provided at the patient's bedside. If the patient is in a nonprivate room, the psychologist may request that the roommate leave until the session is over and then close the door. If the roommate is also bedridden or refuses to leave the room, the session may be conducted (with the roommate's consent) by drawing the curtain around the bed to provide some privacy. Nursing staff are notified so that they know where the patient can be found and so that they do not interrupt the session.... Patients are consulted regarding their comfort with privacy arrangements prior to a treatment session, and every effort is made to accommodate their wishes.

Additionally, clinicians must be aware of facility, state, and Federal regulations involving privacy (Lichtenberg et al., 1998). These standards emphasize the need in some instances to be creative in order maximize the privacy of residents.

To address his concerns about testing, Brian reviews the *Standards for Educational and Psychological Testing* (American Educational Research Association, American Psychological Association, National Council on Measurement in Education, 1999). He learns that tests should be administered according to standardized procedures and, when exceptions must be made, the departure from standardized administration should be documented, including the nature of the departure and the reason for the departure (Standards 5.1 and 5.2). In general, to obtain valid results, the testing environment should be reasonably comfortable, with minimal distractions, similar to the conditions under which the test was standardized and the norms and interpretive data were obtained (Standard 5.4). He also considers the information about the use of test scores and normative data (Standard 4, Scales, Norms, and Score Comparability), which was of particular interest because of Mr. A's 6th grade education; specifically, with the MMSE, Brian found that educational level can have a significant impact on the interpretation of tests scores (Folstein, Folstein, & McHugh, 2002). Although not bound by the American Psychological Association's (2002a) Ethics Code, he found the section on testing (ES 9, Assessment) to be very informative.

CONSIDER PERSONAL BELIEFS AND VALUES

Brian believes strongly in the principle of autonomy and wants all competent residents to make decisions about who is present during clinical interviews, testing, and treatment. He believes that it is his responsibility to help Mr. A understand the potential benefits and risks associated with having others present while sensitive personal matters are discussed and with having distractions present during testing, so that Mr. A can make choices about when and how to help Brian help him. Brian also values his role in the treatment team and wants to ensure that those who are providing care and treatment have the information that they need to best serve Mr. A.

Brian again speaks with his supervisor. She confirms that he reviewed the relevant resources and seemed to have an adequate understanding of the issues to make sound choices about how to proceed.

DEVELOP POSSIBLE SOLUTIONS TO THE PROBLEM

Brian realizes that his prior interactions involving Mr. A should have been handled differently, particularly from the perspective of privacy and confidentiality. Going forward, he considers the following options:

1. Return to Mr. A's room, apologize for the interruption, address questions to Mr. A rather than his family, and complete the interview and GDS but not the MMSE because of the

confusion about its interpretation with persons with only 6 years of education.

2. Return to Mr. A's room, ask his roommate's wife to leave for a few minutes, turn up the television so that his roommate is unable to hear the discussion, draw the curtain around Mr. A's bed, and speak softly to Mr. A. Ask Mr. A's wife and son to remain quiet and unobtrusive unless asked a question. Discuss the privacy and testing concerns with Mr. A. and seek his consent to continue with the interview and testing.

3. Inform the nursing staff that Mr. A will be occupied for a little while and that it will be important to have privacy. Return to Mr. A's room, explain to Mr. A and his family and to his roommate and his roommate's wife that additional time with Mr. A is needed and that, because privacy is important, everyone except the roommate will need to leave the room. Explain all of the privacy and testing concerns with Mr. A and seek his consent to continue. Complete the interview and testing.

4. Wait until the next day when there is a better chance of finding Mr. A alone before completing the psychosocial history and testing.

CONSIDER THE POTENTIAL CONSEQUENCES OF VARIOUS SOLUTIONS

1. Brian determines that the first possible solution does not adequately address privacy and confidentiality issues and, by extension, may not result in valid responses to interview questions and the GDS.

2. Brian determines that the second option improves privacy and confidentiality with regard to Mr. A's roommate and his roommate's wife, but not with regard to Mr. A's family—again with the possible result of not obtaining fully forthright and valid responses from Mr. A.

3. The third option addresses privacy and confidentiality issues to the extent possible and maximizes the likelihood of obtaining

honest and valid responses from Mr. A for both interview questions and test items. Clarification may be necessary to help Mr. A's family understand the need for them to leave the room. The importance of their involvement in Mr. A's psychosocial care may need to be emphasized, so that they do not feel excluded and their opinions undervalued.

4. Option four may be appropriate depending on the urgency of the team's need for the information that Brian will obtain. If an additional 15 hours will not make a significant difference, waiting may help to obviate some of the present ethical concerns. However, Brian's facility requires that his intake interviews be completed the day of admission. In addition, the potential exists that the same issues will be encountered the following day, in which case nothing will have been gained by waiting.

CHOOSE AND IMPLEMENT A COURSE OF ACTION

After careful consideration of the possible options, Brian elects to pursue option 3. He confirms with his supervisor that his choice is appropriate.

ASSESS THE OUTCOME AND IMPLEMENT CHANGES AS NEEDED

Brian elicits the support of the nursing staff in helping to maintain privacy. He then returns to Mr. A's room and finds Mr. A's family and his roommate's wife to be understanding. Privacy and confidentiality are maximized. Brian considers the information obtained and test results to be valid, although he still has concerns about the possible effect of the noise from the roommates' television on the attention and memory components of the MMSE, resulting in his decision to readminister the test at the earliest opportunity that a quiet environment can be ensured. Mr. A gives his consent to have his wife and son fully involved in sharing and receiving information, and they do so in a manner that facilitates his psychosocial, nursing, and medical care. No changes were needed.

DISCUSSION

Limitations on privacy and confidentiality and the implications of those limitations for mental health practice are primary concerns in many organizational settings. This case is intended to help readers apply the ethical decision-making model and appreciate its value when anticipating or resolving ethical challenges such as those examined in this case. Although real-world outcomes are not always as ideal as the outcome depicted here, application of the decision-making model can help assure that selected courses of action are based on sound reasoning and appropriate resources.

Conducting mental health evaluations in skilled nursing facilities, hospitals, and other institutional settings provides many challenges that extend well beyond the clinical importance of asking the right question, administering the right tests in appropriate ways, and making accurate interpretations and use of the information obtained. Clinicians must be able negotiate the organizational milieu to meet the needs of all concerned parties. This ability often requires a degree of professional flexibility because of the frequent changes in patients and their families and unit staff. Additionally transitions involving facility administration and professional and legal standards may require adjustments on the part of the clinician.

Learning Exercise

1. What would have been the best way for Brian to handle the situation from the outset?

Ethical Issues and Case Illustrations

PART
II

Professional Competence

CASE 2

A neuropsychologist is hired by a practice that is co-owned by a psychiatrist and a mental health counselor. The practice primarily treats adults. Shortly after joining the practice, she is asked to evaluate a 76-year-old African American man, Mr. B, to determine his ability to continue driving. He has lived alone since the death of his wife 8 years before. His medical history includes congestive heart failure and cognitive problems, as well as pharmacologic treatment of depression that began following the loss of his wife. Despite limited experience with older adults, the neuropsychologist, desiring to please her new employers, agrees to see Mr. B.

After taking a thorough history, the neuropsychologist begins administration of her standard 4-hour test battery. As the testing progresses, Mr. B appears increasingly anxious and angry and seems to be less invested in completing the tests. The neuropsychologist, having completed tests of psychomotor speed and executive functioning, believes she has enough information to make a determination regarding Mr. B's ability to drive. However, she thinks that if, after she has a chance to review the literature on the relationship between neuropsychological test performances and driving, she needs to administer additional tests, she will need to ask Mr. B to return on another day to complete the testing.

Based on Mr. B's reaction to the testing, she is concerned that he would not return at another time. She wonders whether she should persist with the testing now, so that she can have as much information as possible upon which to base her clinical decisions. She is unsure how to proceed. She suggests to Mr. B that they take a brief break, during which she plans to consider her options.

IDENTIFY THE PROBLEM

The neuropsychologist realizes that she is not adequately prepared to handle the current situation. She must decide whether to continue with the evaluation, given her limited experience with geriatric patients and her inadequate knowledge about which tests or other evaluation procedures, if any, will help her to determine whether Mr. B should be driving.

Consider the Significance of the Context and Setting

In the mental health group practice, the neuropsychologist is without immediate access to a neuropsychology colleague who could offer advice or possibly take over the evaluation. However, in contrast to many medical settings where such colleagues are available, there was less urgency to complete the evaluation in 1 day. Nevertheless, if Mr. B is unsafe to drive, each day behind the wheel could place Mr. B and others in danger.

DETERMINE PATIENT AND FAMILY/CAREGIVER ASSETS AND LIMITATIONS

Mr. B has been able to live independently and has driven safely for many years. Although his psychiatrist is concerned about his driving, no family members or friends are available to describe Mr. B's driving behaviors, and no one is available to provide transportation in the event that Mr. B eventually loses his license.

CONSIDER OBLIGATIONS OWED

The neuropsychologist felt an obligation to her new employers to accept a referral that she was not qualified to undertake. However, at present, she believes she has a greater obligation to Mr. B, to ensure that correct clinical decisions are made, given their potential effect on his life and independence.

IDENTIFY AND UTILIZE ETHICAL AND LEGAL RESOURCES

The neuropsychologist understands the ethical and legal guidelines that are relevant to her dilemma. In a recent continuing education course on psychological ethics, she reviewed the American Psychological Association's (APA) Ethics Code (2002a), the Association of State and Provincial Psychology Boards (ASPPB) Code of Conduct (2005), the Standards for Educational and Psychological Testing (SEPT; American Educational Research Association, American Psychological Association, National Council on measurement in Education, 1999), and state laws related to professional competence. Aware that these resources were fairly consistent regarding the issues relevant to this case, she reflects on the relevant sections of the APA Ethics Code for guidance.

The neuropsychologist realizes that she lacks adequate education, training, and experience to perform geriatric evaluations and should not have accepted this referral (Standard 2.01, Boundaries of Competence). However, having accepted the referral, she knows that she must resolve the situation in a manner consistent with Mr. B's best interests.

As she decides whether to proceed with the evaluation at the present time, the neuropsychologist confronts ethical dilemmas and questions related to beneficence and nonmaleficence (General

Principle A). Specifically, if she discontinues the evaluation, will she have sufficient information to answer the referral question that is intended to keep Mr. B and others safe from harm (Ethical Standard 3.04, Avoiding Harm)? Conversely, is there a greater possibility of promoting safety if she renders an opinion regarding Mr. B's ability to drive based on the data that she has already collected (Ethical Standards 9.01, Bases for Assessments; 9.02, Use of Assessments; 9.06, Interpreting Assessment Results)? Although the neuropsychologist may consider conferring with her employers, their lack of expertise in geriatric neuropsychology limits their ability to be of assistance. Consultation with an experienced geriatric neuropsychologist would likely help the neuropsychologist determine an appropriate course of action.

CONSIDER PERSONAL BELIEFS AND VALUES

The neuropsychologist understands that her desire to please her new employers influenced her decision to accept a referral that she was not competent to handle. She also realizes that her preference to err on the side of caution regarding Mr. B's dangerousness, if inadequately supported, could result in a loss of independence that could adversely impact his quality of life and increase his depression (General Principle E, Respect for People's Rights and Dignity).

DEVELOP POSSIBLE SOLUTIONS TO THE PROBLEM

The neuropsychologist realizes that, because of Mr. B's declining investment in the testing, the evaluation cannot be continued at that time. She also suspects that the referral question likely cannot be adequately addressed based on the data collected to that point. She considers the following courses of action: (1) reschedule the remainder of the evaluation for another day, while obtaining supervision from a qualified colleague in the interim; or (2) refer Mr. B to a qualified neuropsychologist, although he may not pursue the referral given his initial experience with the testing.

CONSIDER THE POTENTIAL CONSEQUENCES OF VARIOUS SOLUTIONS

Given her competence with younger adults, the neuropsychologist considers that she may be able to salvage the evaluation by obtaining consultation from a qualified colleague. This course of action would eliminate the need for Mr. B to begin another evaluation, enhance her professional skills, and satisfy her new employers. However, rescheduling the remainder of the test administration may result in a lost opportunity, because Mr. B may not return. Additionally, postponing the evaluation until she is able to obtain adequate consultation could prove harmful to Mr. B or others by delaying the identification of any safety concerns.

In contrast, referring Mr. B to a qualified neuropsychologist would ensure that an appropriate evaluation was performed and that appropriate decisions were made regarding the Mr. B's safety and independence. She could provide the geriatric neuropsychologist with the information obtained during the clinical interview and the test data already obtained, so that redundant efforts and unnecessary additional time could be avoided. However, Mr. B would need to present for another evaluation session, and he seemed unlikely to do so. In addition, the esteem of the neuropsychologist's employers and colleagues may be adversely affected.

CHOOSE AND IMPLEMENT A COURSE OF ACTION

The neuropsychologist decided that it would be in Mr. B's best interest to be referred to a qualified geriatric neuropsychologist. When they returned from the break, she informed Mr. B of the need for the referral and gave him the name and contact information for a geriatric neuropsychologist in the area. Mr. B seemed relieved that he would not have to do any more testing that day, but he was angry that he had been put through such testing for what appeared to be no reason. He stated that he would continue the testing with another clinician at another time, but the neuropsychologist was not convinced. Additionally, with Mr. B's authorization (Ethical Standard 4.05, Disclosures) she contacted the geriatric neuropsychologist to discuss the particulars of the case.

ASSESS THE OUTCOME AND IMPLEMENT CHANGES AS NEEDED

A subsequent follow-up call to the geriatric neuropsychologist revealed that Mr. B had not followed through with the referral. The original neuropsychologist placed calls to Mr. B to encourage him to complete the evaluation, but she was unable to reach him, and he did not return her calls. She eventually provided her recommendations in a letter to Mr. B. Mr. B's next few sessions with the psychiatrist were spent complaining about the neuropsychologist and the testing. He then missed a couple of sessions, stopped coming, and was not heard from again. Calls and letters to Mr. B's home received no reply.

The psychiatrist, mental health counselor, and neuropsychologist met to discuss the case. The neuropsychologist was reassured that she need not accept any referrals that she was not qualified to examine or treat. They all agreed to keep the communication between them open, so that similar situations would be less likely to occur in the future. They were all disappointed that they could not do more to help Mr. B.

DISCUSSION

Professional competence is based on the general bioethical principles of nonmaleficence and beneficence. To minimize the potential for harming patients and maximize the potential for helping patients, clinicians must possess the requisite specialized knowledge and skills to perform the requested services. Professional competence in a mental health discipline is obtained through a combination of education, supervised training, and experience. Competence in a subspecialty, such as geriatric mental health, requires additional specialized knowledge and supervised experience. Thus, competence in geriatric mental health consists of three main components: competence in mental health, competence in gerontology, and competence in the integration of mental health and gerontology.

Competent mental health practitioners have adequate education, training, and experience in the fundamental activities of their discipline, including obtaining and reviewing relevant background information, conducting clinical interviews, using various assessment measures, providing treatment of the patient and/or family members, and consulting with other service providers as needed. In addition to the core competencies of a mental health discipline, competent geriatric mental health professionals have appropriate education, training, and experience in gerontology.

Late adulthood represents a distinct developmental stage, with unique issues and concerns. Clinicians working with the elderly must be familiar with the unique issues of the asymptomatic members of the aging population, and they must possess an in-depth understanding of the psychopathology of the elderly and various treatment options, including psychological, pharmacologic, and rehabilitative options. Additionally, familiarity with the more common medical disorders experienced by the elderly and the potential psychological side effects of the medications used to treat them is essential. Depending on the nature of services provided, geriatric mental health professionals may also need to acquire a thorough understanding of the neuropathology of the elderly. Such understanding includes knowledge of how the neuropathology, as well as the psychopathology, evidenced by the elderly translates into performance on measures of cognitive and psychological functioning. Geriatric mental health professionals should be able to discuss these issues with appropriate parties and to make referrals as needed. The ability to do so requires the ability to integrate competence in mental health services, gerontology, and the psychopathology and neuropathology of the elderly. Competent mental health assessment and treatment of the elderly must be specific to the population to whom, and the setting in which, services are offered.

Competence in a mental health discipline is readily identified through certification, licensure, and, if relevant, board certification. In addition to board certification, competence in geriatrics may, depending on the discipline, be further determined through additional formal peer review in the form of added qualifications.

Competence is not a static trait. Attainment of competence at one point in a career does not guarantee that the clinician will maintain competence in the years to come. Rapid advances are being made in geriatric medicine, neuroimaging, and other areas of relevance to geriatric mental health, and clinicians have a responsibility to remain abreast of emerging information.

In addition to being competent to perform clinical activities, complete professional competence requires education, supervised training, and experience in anticipating and negotiating ethical challenges. Because of the complex biopsychosocial circumstances in which many elderly patients present for mental health services, ethical competence is as important as clinical competence. Clinicians have a fundamental responsibility to seek continuing education and consultation on the ethical and legal aspects of their practices, and particularly when changing practice contexts.

Unfortunately, there seems to be a shortage of geriatric mental health professionals (Rosen, 2005), and the shortage may increase as the U.S. population ages, unless a concerted effort is made to increase training opportunities, which will require increased allocation of funds for this purpose. For example, the National Association of Social Workers (NASW) is facing a shortage of competent geriatric clinicians (NASW, 2006a). As a result, NASW has recommended the establishment of scholarships and loan forgiveness programs to encourage social workers to become specialized in gerontological social work (NASW, 2006b). The NASW also recommended that social workers receive continuing education opportunities related to serving older adults.

The future availability of qualified geriatric psychologists and psychiatrists is similarly bleak. With only 3% of psychologists identifying geriatrics as their primary area of practice (Rosen, 2005), a shortage of geropsychologists already exists, and recent Federal grant cuts portend serious problems for older adults in need of psychological services in the future (Clay, 2006).

Geriatric psychiatry is facing problems of a different kind. In its most recent *Status of Geriatrics Workforce Study*, the Association of Directors of Geriatric Academic Programs (ADGAP; 2007) reported that, as of April, 2007 there were 1,596 board certified geriatric psychiatrists in the United States. That is, there was one board certified geropsychiatrist for every 11,372 older Americans, and the ADGAP projected that the ratio will decrease to one geropsychiatrist for every 20,195 Americans age 75 and older by the year 2030. Unlike social work, however, there are plenty of available geriatric psychiatry fellowship training slots for interested applicants. For the academic year 2006–2007, 136 geriatric psychiatry fellowship first-year training slots were available, but only 68 (50%) were filled. In 2007, 24 physicians (MD) educated in the United States entered geriatric psychiatry fellowship programs, which is less than 0.2 % of all U.S. medical students who graduated in 2007. This number also represents a decrease from 30 in 2003. The remainder of the geropsychiatry fellows were from foreign medical schools. The low number of geriatric psychiatrists has been attributed to members of the specialty earning significantly less income and having less predictable work schedules than physicians in other medical and surgical specialties (American Geriatrics Society, 2008).

In the case of Mr. B, the neuropsychologist may have been competent to practice in her discipline, but not in the specialty of geriatrics. Geriatric neuropsychologists are frequently asked to determine the ability of older adults to drive safely and therefore are aware of the inherent limitations of using neuropsychological tests alone to make such determinations (Reger & Welsh, 2004). The neuropsychologist in the present case did not seem prepared to address this complex issue appropriately.

Additionally, the interaction of Mr. B's race and cultural background, his age, and the neuropsychological evaluation context was not adequately considered. Some African American older adults do not have the same degree of confidence in health care providers as do younger adults or members of the dominant culture, which can lead to increased anxiety and defensiveness in the presence of health care professionals (Byrd & Manly, 2005). Such feelings can ultimately affect the results of the neuropsychological evaluation, particularly if the clinician is not aware of the issues and is not prepared to take steps to minimize the impact of the issues on the validity of the results. Thus, by overstepping boundaries of competence, clinicians may provide detrimental services in unanticipated and unintended ways.

Learning Exercises

1. Describe a course of education and training that you would recommend to someone who is considering entering your discipline and is interested in specializing in geriatrics.

2. List three specific steps that you would take to ensure your competence if you were to change work settings, such as transitioning from a skilled nursing facility to a private practice.

7 Human Relations

Dr. C is a psychiatrist who has a practice in a rural community and consults in nursing facilities in the area. In recent weeks, a patient of many years, 78-year-old Mr. Seer, has been unable to pay his insurance co-pays. Dr. C is more concerned about Mr. Seer's financial situation than the co-pays, and she asks whether there are any financial problems. Mr. Seer reports that he has recently fallen in love and has been giving gifts to his new "fiancé" but is rather circumspect about the details. Less than a week later, Dr. C receives a frantic phone call from Mr. Seer's closest relative, a niece, stating that Mr. Seer had depleted his savings of more than $80,000 in the past 3 weeks at the instruction of his new friend, Roberta. The niece begs Dr. C to convince Mr. Seer to stop giving Roberta his money or to deem him "incompetent" to make financial decisions for himself. When Dr. C hears the name "Roberta," she thinks "Oh no." Roberta is known by professionals in local nursing facilities to "befriend" men in the facilities and encourage them to share their ATM and credit cards, and she often finds her way into their wills, much to the shock and dismay of family members. Dr. C is determined not to let Mr. Seer and his family be victimized by Roberta, and wonders whether she should tell Roberta to seek romance elsewhere.

IDENTIFY THE PROBLEM

Dr. C's patient, Mr. Seer, seems to have been persuaded by his new fiancé to make financial decisions that may not be in his best interest. Dr. C feels a responsibility to protect her patient from probable victimization by the fiancé. However, Mr. Seer seems happier than he has been in a long time, and he may be deriving considerable emotional benefit, at least for the time being, from his relationship with his fiancé. Dr. C, also feeling some pressure from Mr. Seer's niece, considers how she should intervene, not wanting to violate confidentiality and lacking evidence to characterize Mr. Seer as lacking the cognitive capacity to make financial decisions for himself.

CONSIDER THE SIGNIFICANCE OF THE CONTEXT AND SETTING

Dr. C treats Mr. Seer in her private practice. However, she has additional information about Mr. Seer's fiancé from her consultation in skilled nursing facilities. Dr. C is bound by confidentiality requirements to not discuss Mr. Seer with his fiancé, family members, or others without his permission. At the same time, however, she is concerned that Mr. Seer has been harmed financially and will likely suffer, both financially and emotionally, because of his relationship with his fiancé. Because treatment occurs in a private practice setting, Dr. C does not have the direct support or assistance of other professionals, which she would have in many organizational settings.

DETERMINE PATIENT AND FAMILY/CAREGIVER ASSETS AND LIMITATIONS

Mr. Seer's niece seems to be one of the only people who can help Mr. Seer avoid further victimization. However, she may be as invested in preserving her own inheritance as she is in Mr. Seer's interests.

CONSIDER OBLIGATIONS OWED

Dr. C's primary obligation is to provide the psychiatric services for which Mr. Seer seeks treatment. Mr. Seer has not identified his relationship with his fiancé as a problem or a focus of treatment. Nevertheless, broadly conceptualized, she should help Mr. Seer to clarify an issue of emerging importance (financial problems) and to anticipate situations that may be emotionally and pragmatically detrimental to Mr. Seer in the future. Dr. C does not have an obligation to assist Mr. Seer's niece in the pursuit of her goals.

IDENTIFY AND UTILIZE ETHICAL AND LEGAL RESOURCES

Dr. C considers confidentiality requirements as detailed by professional ethics and state law (American Psychiatric Association, 2006, Section 4). Because Mr. Seer has not been deemed incompetent and there was previously no reason to question his judgment or decision-making capacity, he is the holder of privilege and Dr. C cannot even acknowledge that he is her patient without his consent. However, Dr. C also knows that she has clinical and ethical responsibilities to serve her patients in ways that are beneficial (beneficence) and to help them, when possible, avoid being harmed by others. Unsure about which ethical obligations and resources should be considered primary, she contacts the American Psychiatric Association's (APA) ethics committee for advice.

CONSIDER PERSONAL BELIEFS AND VALUES

Dr. C appreciates her responsibility to maintain confidentiality, but her primary value is that she should protect her patient from further financial ruin and emotional distress. She does not believe that Mr. Seer's relationship with his fiancé is healthy or in his best interests. She also believes that Roberta has victimized too many vulnerable men already and does not want to witness her patient being victimized when she can help stop it.

DEVELOP POSSIBLE SOLUTIONS TO THE PROBLEM

Dr. C considers the following options:

1. Inform Mr. Seer of Roberta's history of establishing relationships with elderly men and taking their money, and encourage him to end the relationship.
2. Confront Roberta when their paths next cross in a nursing home and advise her to end the relationship or she will be reported to Adult Protective Services.
3. Advise Mr. Seer's niece to handle the situation by discussing her concerns with Mr. Seer, confronting Roberta, and/or reporting the matter to Adult Protective Services.
4. Help Mr. Seer, in the therapeutic context, examine his relationship with his fiancé, including both the benefits and potential risks associated with the relationship, and assist him with making life decisions that he deems best.

CONSIDER THE POTENTIAL CONSEQUENCES OF VARIOUS SOLUTIONS

Dr. C identifies and considers the following possible consequences of each of the possible solutions:

1. Informing Mr. Seer of Roberta's history may result in Mr. Seer ending the relationship or setting limits with Roberta regarding the sharing of money. However, this option also may be emotionally distressing to Mr. Seer, perceived as inappropriately meddlesome, and met with defensiveness, including the possibility that Mr. Seer will terminate treatment.
2. By confronting Roberta about her relationship with Mr. Seer, Dr. C would be violating patient confidentiality and trust. Also,

the potential for such action to affect Roberta's behavior is unknown, but may very well not be helpful.

3. The nature of the relationship between Mr. Seer and his niece is unclear, as is the extent to which he may be influenced by his niece. Additionally, discussing Mr. Seer with his niece, in the absence of appropriate authorization, would violate confidentiality and could adversely affect the therapeutic relationship.

4. Helping Mr. Seer to more closely and thoughtfully examine his relationship with his fiancé and explore his choices has the potential to reinforce or alter Mr. Seer's current choices and is respectful of his autonomy.

CHOOSE AND IMPLEMENT A COURSE OF ACTION

Dr. C chooses option 4, facilitating Mr. Seer's examination of his thoughts, feelings, and choices regarding his relationship with his fiancé, so that he can best weigh the benefits and risks associated with the relationship.

ASSESS THE OUTCOME AND IMPLEMENT CHANGES AS NEEDED

Mr. Seer discusses in therapy sessions his relationship with his fiancé. He is happier than he has been in years and clearly states that he intends for Roberta to have access to all of his assets, now and in the future, stating, "She's earned it." He further indicated that his niece and other extended family members had never been particularly involved in his life, and he felt no obligation to give them anything.

Dr. C continues to believe that her patient is being victimized and feels angry, frustrated, and helpless that she cannot do more to protect him. She considered making an anonymous call to Adult Protective Services but doubts that they would be able to intervene. She did refer Mr. Seer for neuropsychological testing to clarify his decision-making capacity, but he would not pursue the testing. When Mr. Seer's niece called back, Dr. C informed her that she should talk to Mr. Seer directly. The niece reported that she tried to talk to her uncle, but he refused to talk about Roberta and hung up on her. The niece then yelled at Dr. C, calling her a "quack shrink" for not doing more about the situation, and hung up on her.

DISCUSSION

The "sweetheart scam" has long been one way that older adults have been victimized by others preying on their vulnerabilities, such as loneliness. However, it is discriminatory to assume that the older adult, simply because of age, cannot "see through" the scam and make an informed choice about the relationship and dispersion of finances. As with other types of individual differences, such as race, gender, religion, disability, sexual orientation, and socioeconomic status, mental health professionals must not engage in unfair discrimination based on the patient's age. Mental health professionals must respect the autonomous decision making of competent older adults just as with younger adults. Despite the unique issues often experienced by many geriatric patients, it is advisable for clinicians to avoid making assumptions based solely on the age of their patients. Failure to appropriately consider the ability of older patients to solve problems reflects a lack of appreciation of their right to be involved in discussions that may have substantial implications for their independence, treatment, and care.

Many older adults who pursue or receive mental health services have family members, caregivers, friends, and/or other health care professionals who are interested or invested in the older adult's mental health care. Such persons may pay for services, provide transportation, help provide background information, or provide some other type of assistance or support, resulting in a perceived or legitimate entitlement to some degree of direct involvement in the older adult's mental health evaluation and/or treatment. It can be tempting for clinicians to turn to such persons for assistance with complex or difficult patients. Similarly, clinicians may experience internal or external pressure to provide supportive counseling services to others involved in the patient's life. These situations can raise sensitive clinical and ethical issues involving multiple relationships and confidentiality that must be explored carefully with all parties during the informed consent process or as early in the course of evaluation or treatment as possible. Geriatric mental health professionals should refrain from entering into multiple relationships that may reasonably be expected to reduce their effectiveness in providing services to the older adult client. In many situations in which multiple relationships develop, conflicts of interest may arise, requiring the clinician to pit obligations owed to one person against those owed to another person, resulting in the interests of at least one person being sacrificed.

It is common for the adult children of older adults to seek mental health services for their parents. Referrals may also come from other health care professionals, attorneys, agencies, institutions, and others. Geriatric mental professionals have an obligation to cooperate with other professionals to serve the older adult patient most effectively. Third-party requests for mental health services at times involve some degree of misinformation or subterfuge to get the older adult into the treatment setting. When requests for services come from a third party, clinicians must clarify with all parties at the outset the nature of the roles and relationships of all parties, the services that will be provided, payment arrangements, and dissemination of information. Competent older adults must be involved in this process and voluntarily consent to the arrangements.

Many geriatric mental health professionals are receiving increased numbers of forensic (i.e., legal) referrals, such as those to address financial decision-making capacity, and this trend is likely to continue. "The incidence of cases in which capacity is an issue will increase substantially in the coming years because of the aging demographic bulge and because of the greater incidence of dementia that accompanies the aging process" (p. 1), and "the failure to assess a client's capacity has been asserted as grounds for legal malpractice by would-be beneficiaries of a client's largess" (p. 2) (American Bar Association Commission on Law and Aging & American Psychological Association, 2005).

COOPERATION WITH OTHER PROFESSIONALS

Geriatric mental health professions frequently provide services in a multidisciplinary context. The appropriate treatment of medical, neurological, and/or psychiatric influences on cognitive and emotional functioning frequently requires contributions from a variety of medical professionals. Mental health professionals have a responsibility to facilitate necessary evaluations and treatment or to cooperate with such professionals if the multidisciplinary services are already under way. Such consultation should be performed with sensitivity to confidentiality issues. For example, mental health clinicians do not share with colleagues personal information about a patient that was obtained in the course of an evaluation or treatment that is not pertinent to the services being provided by the other professional.

INSTITUTIONAL PRACTICE

Geriatric mental health professionals often perform services as consultants to, or employees of, institutions. Such institutions include community-based settings, such as senior centers or home-based services; outpatient settings, such as mental health or primary care clinics; day treatment or partial hospital programs; inpatient medical, psychiatric, or rehabilitation hospitals; and long-term care settings, such as skilled nursing facilities and assisted living centers (American Psychological Association Presidential Task Force on the Assessment of Age-Consistent Memory Decline and Dementia, 1998). Clinicians should be aware that patients' levels of independence and functional ability are likely to vary among settings, and different clinical practices may be required in each setting. In addition, variations on the ethical obligations owed may occur across settings.

Consistent with the principle of autonomy and the right of individuals to accept or decline services, clinicians have a responsibility before services are provided and as needed after services have commenced to establish the parameters of proposed services with all relevant parties. Clinicians also must (a) clarify with all parties who the client will be (e.g., the identified patient, a couple, an attorney, or an institution) and what the clinician's role will be with the client and other involved parties, (b) provide information about the purpose and nature of the proposed services, (c) describe the probable uses of information obtained and who will have access to the information, and (d) clarify limits of confidentiality. If jurisdictional laws or organizational rules prohibit the provision of such information, involved persons are informed accordingly. Knowledge of the financing and reimbursement systems that govern the operations of the facilities in which one works is an aspect of professional competence because of the potential for such factors to affect service delivery or patient financial responsibility.

Conflicts may arise between the best interests of the older adult and the needs or interests of the staff or management of the institution in which the services are provided. Although ethical challenges are best resolved by serving the best interests of the patient, it may be difficult to establish the best interests of the patient when the patient lacks the cognitive capacity to assist with such determinations, and professionals disagree. Determination of *best interests* requires a comparative assessment made by one person for another who is unable to make that determination independently (Beauchamp & Childress, 2001).

To promote the best interests of a patient, the clinician must make a quality-of-life determination, selecting the option that offers the greatest benefit from among those available. The clinician, in an attempt to protect the patient's well-being, must assess the risks and benefits of various options, taking into consideration the patient's comfort level and potential restoration or loss of function. Best-interest determinations may range from the most serious questions, such as those involving life sustaining efforts and procedures, to the relatively minor. For example, consider the case of 88-year-old man with depressed mood, memory problems, and a tendency to confabulate who resides in a skilled nursing facility. During one psychotherapy session, he informs you that a staff member grabbed and twisted his finger during the night, causing considerable pain but no obvious injury or reduction in movement. However, he does not recall which staff member was involved in the incident. He is afraid to notify the nursing or medical staff of the incident because of fear of retaliation from the staff member involved. He worries that retaliation may take the form of additional painful incidents or simply a lack of care or attention when he needs assistance with eating or toileting. He instructs you to not mention the incident to anyone. You are torn between your due diligence to report or investigate the matter in the interest of protecting the patient, and your obligation to maintain confidentiality. Complicating matters are the fact that the patient may be confabulating and your difficulty in determining what steps you could take that would help to protect the patient, given that fear of staff retaliation, however rare, is not necessarily a sign of paranoia.

Making best-interest determinations for another is a great responsibility and should, to the extent possible, be based on an understanding of the patient's values and preferences. Family members and prior documentation from the patient, such as advance directives, may be of considerable value in this process. Conflicts between ethics and organizational demands should be clarified, with a commitment to professional ethics being emphasized and an attempt made to resolve the conflict in a manner that is consistent with high standards of ethical practice.

Learning Exercise

1.   You work in a hospital where an 81-year-old woman has been admitted because of diabetes-related gangrene in her legs. Her surgeon has told her that unless she undergoes bilateral above-the-knee amputations, she will die soon. When she refuses to undergo the surgery, the surgeon asks you to "go talk some sense into her." He then states, "If she continues to refuse, document her incompetence to make such decisions." You find her to be cognitively intact. What do you do with regard to the patient? What do you do with regard to the surgeon?

8 Privacy, Confidentiality, and Informed Consent

Mr. Jones, 79 years old, widowed, and living alone is referred for psychotherapy by his psychiatrist as part of a comprehensive multidisciplinary intervention approach to early stage dementia of the Alzheimer's type. The various health care and mental health professionals are not part of the same group, working instead within separate practices in the region. Mr. Jones is brought for an initial interview by his daughter. He is legally competent to make all of the decisions that govern his life, including providing consent to treatment. Mr. Jones authorizes the psychotherapist to discuss his case, including the results of any testing of mood or cognition, with his daughter.

The clinical interview revealed that Mr. Jones has a rocky relationship with his son, and he suspects that his son wants his home and money. Nevertheless, Mr. Jones relies on his son for maintenance around the house and for transportation. Mr. Jones arrives for a subsequent psychotherapy session with his son. The psychotherapist invites Mr. Jones into the office, at which point the son says, "You want me in there too, right, Dad?" Mr. Jones, looking uncomfortable, says, "Uh, ya, I guess." At that moment, the psychotherapist's secretary informs him that the psychiatrist is on the phone. The psychotherapist excuses himself and takes the call to find the psychiatrist stating, "I'm hoping you can update me on Mr. Jones' emotional state and family dynamics."

IDENTIFY THE PROBLEM(S)

Mr. Jones' son and psychiatrist are asking for involvement in, and information about, Mr. Jones' mental health care. There may be some value in having a joint session with Mr. Jones and his son, and Mr. Jones' overall mental health treatment goals will likely be well served through open dialogue between practitioners; however, issues of privacy and confidentiality, the emotional security of the therapeutic environment, and other clinical issues must be considered.

CONSIDER THE SIGNIFICANCE OF THE CONTEXT AND SETTING

Mr. Jones' lives independently and is competent to make decisions for himself. Although he has a strained relationship with his son and is suspicious of his son's motives, he relies on his son for certain types of assistance. Because of this partial dependence on his son, he may feel obligated to grant his son greater access into his personal matters, including psychotherapy, than he would prefer. His hesitancy in responding to his son's request to attend the therapy session supports this position.

In the context of multidisciplinary treatment, discussion among professionals is essential for Mr. Jones' welfare. However, because the treatment occurs on an outpatient basis with professionals who practice independently of each other, a universally applied consent form was not used. Instead each clinician was responsible for identifying, clarifying, and addressing foreseeable issues related to the exchange of information prior to rendering services.

DETERMINE PATIENT AND FAMILY/CAREGIVER ASSETS AND LIMITATIONS

Mr. Jones has some relatively mild cognitive deficits but is still competent to make decisions for himself in all areas of his life. However, he is dependent on others for transportation and assistance with aspects of home life, and his dependence will increase over time. Mr. Jones' son is involved in his father's life, and the psychotherapist's initial impression is that the son is caring and supportive. The psychotherapist does not know whether Mr. Jones' suspicion of his son's motives is valid or perhaps associated with the suspiciousness that is commonly experienced by persons who are forgetful, particularly those who may not have been the most trusting of people throughout their lives. Mr. Jones' daughter seems to be supportive and has Mr. Jones' trust, although she may not be as accessible as his son.

CONSIDER OBLIGATIONS OWED

The psychotherapist's primary obligation is to Mr. Jones. However, to be of greatest service to Mr. Jones, obligations also exist to collaborate with the psychiatrist and possibly other professionals involved in Mr. Jones' care, as well as to gather information from and perhaps exchange information with his adult children.

IDENTIFY AND UTILIZE ETHICAL AND LEGAL RESOURCES

According to the psychotherapist's professional ethics code, state laws, numerous scholarly publications, and prior discussions with colleagues, the psychotherapist knows that some degree of family involvement in the treatment process and sharing information with colleagues to promote Mr. Jones' welfare is consistent with the principle of beneficence. However, sharing information without considering Mr. Jones' wishes and obtaining the appropriate written consents constitutes a failure to respect autonomy and may be harmful to the therapeutic alliance and the pursuit of treatment goals.

Specifically, the Code of Ethics of the American Mental Health Counselors Association (2000) addresses the importance of maintaining confidentiality (Principle 2, Clients' Rights, section C; Principle 3, Confidentiality), obtaining Mr. Jones' consent before sharing information with others (Principle 1, Welfare of the Consumer, section J), and collaborating with other professionals such as Mr. Jones psychiatrist (Principle 8, Professional Relationships, section A). The psychotherapist's state laws similarly addressed these issues (Behnke, Perlin, & Bernstein, 2003). Additionally, the *Opinions of the Ethics Committee on The Principles of Medical Ethics with Annotations Especially Applicable to Psychiatry* (American Psychiatric Association, 2001, Section 4-Y) and a variety of scholarly works provided clarification of the psychotherapist's clinical, ethical, and legal responsibilities (e.g., Appelbaum, 2002; Ardern, 2004; Bush & Martin, 2008; Friedland, 1994; Haut & Muehleman, 1986; Smith-Bell & Winslade, 1999).

CONSIDER PERSONAL BELIEFS AND VALUES

The psychotherapist values open communication among parties that have an interest in Mr. Jones' emotional state, believing that such communication will likely promote Mr. Jones' welfare at the present time and particularly as his life progresses. However, the psychotherapist values Mr. Jones' right to privacy and confidentiality and his right to decide who should receive information about his mood and the sensitive issues discussed in psychotherapy.

DEVELOP POSSIBLE SOLUTIONS TO THE PROBLEM

The psychotherapist considers the following solutions:

1. Give the psychiatrist a brief synopsis, and then hold the session with Mr. Jones and his son.

2. Give the psychiatrist a brief synopsis, and then hold the session only with Mr. Jones.
3. Tell the psychiatrist that the case cannot be discussed because of confidentiality issues, and inform the son that he cannot attend the therapy session.
4. Inform the psychiatrist that a session is about to begin and find a good time to return the call. Then meet individually with Mr. Jones, seek his permission to discuss his status with his psychiatrist, and determine whether he really wants his son to be present during the session. Based on Mr. Jones' wishes, either invite the son to attend the session or inform the son that the session will be held only with Mr. Jones.

CONSIDER THE POTENTIAL CONSEQUENCES OF VARIOUS SOLUTIONS

1. Discussing Mr. Jones' status with his psychiatrist without getting his consent (which probably should have been obtained during the initial interview) would violate confidentiality. However, simply refusing to discuss the case with the psychiatrist threatens the spirit of collaboration between professionals that is important with multidisciplinary treatment and may not be in Mr. Jones' best interests.
2. Allowing Mr. Jones' son to attend the session without further clarifying Mr. Jones' wishes could undermine the psychotherapeutic process. However, having his son present may provide important information about their relationship, the accuracy of Mr. Jones' impressions about his son, and the degree to which his son is likely to be helpful in the future.
3. Refusing to discuss the case with the psychiatrist and to involve the son without further determining Mr. Jones' wishes will likely result in adversarial interactions that do not advance Mr. Jones' treatment goals.
4. Informing the psychiatrist that there is not enough time to speak but that you will return the call in a timely manner will likely be acceptable to the psychiatrist and allows time to obtain

consent from Mr. Jones (or to explore any reasons why Mr. Jones would not want his treating clinicians to speak). Taking a few moments to clarify whether Mr. Jones want his son to be present demonstrates respect for Mr. Jones' right to make such decisions, which will likely enhance the therapeutic alliance. His son's reaction to this requirement may also be informative for the psychotherapist.

CHOOSE AND IMPLEMENT A COURSE OF ACTION

The psychotherapist, prepared for such situations, acted in a manner consistent with the last option. That is, the psychiatrist was informed that a session was about to begin (without even acknowledging that Mr. Jones was a patient), and a time was scheduled to return the call. The psychotherapist then asked Mr. Jones' son to wait in the waiting room for a few minutes while just the two of them met, and the son agreed. Mr. Jones readily consented (in writing) for the psychotherapist to speak with the psychiatrist, and he chose to let his son attend the session, although with the understanding that the son's participation would not be a regular occurrence.

ASSESS THE OUTCOME AND IMPLEMENT CHANGES AS NEEDED

The session with Mr. Jones and his son was informative and served to open a relationship between the psychotherapist and Mr. Jones' son that could prove to be important over time. The psychotherapist later discussed the case with the psychiatrist.

DISCUSSION

What I may see or hear in the course of the treatment or even outside of the treatment in regard to the life of men, which on no account one must spread abroad, I will keep to myself, holding such things shameful to be spoken about. Hippocrates[1]

Part of being a competent clinician specializing in geriatric mental health is knowing that persons other than the patient will likely want to exchange information about the patient. The potential involvement of family members, caregivers, companions, and others creates rich opportunities for gathering and exchanging information about the patient, in order to better understand and serve him, but such involvement also increases the potential for violations of the patient's privacy. Advanced knowledge of potentially interested parties allows the clinician to anticipate clinical and ethical challenges that may arise, so that they can be successfully negotiated when they occur. Such is the situation with Mr. Jones. To successfully handle this situation, the psychotherapist should establish a priori the appropriate steps to take from both clinical and ethical perspectives. A proactive approach to anticipating such situations facilitates good decision making when the need arises. Failure to anticipate and prepare for commonly encountered situations such as this tends to lead to awkward interactions and inappropriate decisions.

Although this case was resolved rather easily and optimally, had the psychotherapist not anticipated such a situation and prepared for it in advance, the choices made could have adversely affected Mr. Jones' therapy and mental health care as well as violated professional ethics and laws. Thus, the importance of anticipating potential problems with confidentiality and addressing them during the informed consent process cannot be overstated.

This case also demonstrates the awkwardness that may exist when a clinician from one discipline contacts a clinician from another discipline about a patient. Had the psychotherapist simply refused to discuss the case because of confidentiality requirements, an unpleasant confrontation may have ensued. Multidisciplinary patient care is much easier when a foundation of good will and collaboration has been established and lines of communication are open.

---

[1] From the Hippocratic Oath; translated from Greek by Ludwig Edelstein. Retrieved June 23, 2006 from www.pbs.org/wgbh/nova/doctors/oath_classical.html.

FOUNDATIONS OF TRUST IN TESTING AND TREATMENT

The ability of patients to communicate openly and honestly with clinicians has traditionally served as the foundation of medical and mental health treatment. Patients must feel confident that their innermost thoughts and sensitive aspects of their past can be safely divulged. Trust that the therapist will maintain the privacy of this sensitive information is central in promoting the sincere communication between parties that forms the cornerstone of the therapeutic process. Discussion of the patient's private information outside of the therapeutic context, without the consent of the patient or a designated representative, may destroy the patient's trust, possibly harm the patient in significant ways, and end the patient's willingness to engage in further treatment with any therapist. Patients expect that the information conveyed to mental health professionals will be kept within the therapeutic dyad (Miller & Thelen, 1986). With few exceptions, protecting privacy protects patients. Thus, the importance of protecting patient information in most mental health treatment contexts cannot be overstated, and this importance is reflected in the jurisdictional laws and codes of ethics that govern practice.

Privacy, confidentiality, and privilege are related terms pertaining to the protection of communications from patients to clinicians in a professional context. *Privacy* refers to the right of individuals to choose how much of their personal information may be shared with others. Privacy is a fundamental human right; it is essential to ensure one's dignity and freedom of self-determination (Koocher & Keith-Spiegel, 1998) and is based on the principle of respect for autonomy (Beauchamp & Childress, 2001). *Confidentiality* is based on the right to privacy and poses limits on the release of patient information to others.

Privilege is defined as "a right or immunity granted as a peculiar benefit, advantage, or favor" (Merriam-Webster, 1988, p. 936). Privilege relieves the clinician from having to testify in court about a patient's communications; thus, it is a narrower concept than confidentiality. By *invoking privilege*, the patient can prevent the clinician from testifying or releasing records about intimate personal details

(Behnke, Perlin, & Bernstein, 2003). By *waiving privilege*, the patient allows the clinician to testify or release records in a legal proceeding. Accordingly, privilege belongs to patients and is invoked or waived at their discretion. Without a privilege statute or a common-law rule, the clinician can be charged with contempt of court for refusing to testify about information shared by a patient in a professional context (Smith-Bell & Winslade, 1999).

The willingness of patients to convey information that may render them vulnerable to embarrassment or other harmful consequences is as essential for mental health evaluations as it is for treatment. Diagnostic accuracy and the usefulness of recommendations depend upon the accuracy and completeness of relevant patient information. However, geriatric mental health professionals and their patients face multiple threats to confidentiality (see Table 8.1).

Consistent with intuitive expectations, research indicates that individuals have a reduced willingness to disclose personal information when they are informed that there are limits to confidentiality (Haut & Muehleman, 1986; Nowell & Spruill, 1993; Woods & McNamara,

Table 8.1

EXAMPLES OF THREATS TO CONFIDENTIALITY IN GERIATRIC MENTAL HEALTH PRACTICE

- Practical limitations associated with inpatient and residential settings, such as roommates and staff
- Team approach to evaluation and treatment
- Requests for services by third parties, such as family members, attorneys, or organizations
- Mandated reporting requirements, such as danger to self or others
- Government monitoring of services funded by public payers such as Medicare
- Managed care oversight, including utilization review
- Clinician disclosure to resolve unpaid debts
- Electronic storage and transfer of patient information
- Litigation

The examples listed do not include a patient's or legal representative's request for the clinician to disclose information or a patient's waiver of privilege in litigated matters.

1980), particularly for patients with more severe problems (Taube & Elwork, 1990). In addition, fear of confidentiality infringement reduces the willingness of patients to disclose relevant and necessary information regarding of their personality traits or demographic background (Kremer & Gesten, 1998). As the result of either wishing to facilitate patient openness or an insufficient appreciation of the importance of educating patients about these matters, many clinicians fail to provide full disclosure of the limits of confidentiality (Baird & Rupert, 1987), resulting in inaccurate patient expectations and increased likelihood of an adverse outcome.

LEGAL CONSIDERATIONS

Older adult patients have a legal right to expect adherence to privacy, confidentiality, and privilege until they provide consent for the information to be shared or are deemed incompetent to make such decisions (American Psychological Association, 2004).

A Constitutional Right

The specific rights and restrictions regarding privacy have been established at both the Federal and state levels. Despite the absence of the word *privacy* in the U.S. Constitution, the U.S. Supreme Court has recognized privacy as a constitutional right (*Eisenstadt v. Baird*, 1972; *Griswold v. Connecticut*, 1965; *Hawaii Psychiatric Society v. Ariyoshi*, 1979), reflecting the importance that society has long placed on privacy as a primary value and fundamental right (Bersoff, 1999; Smith-Bell & Winslade, 1999). Nevertheless, the protection of sensitive disclosures by patients is not absolute. Courts have placed limitations on the right to privacy (*Bowers v. Hardwick*, 1985; *Roe v. Wade*, 1973; *Tarasoff v. Regents of the University of California*, 1976; *Whalen v. Roe*, 1976), indicating that, under certain circumstances, the value of human safety, especially for vulnerable individuals such as children and the elderly, outweighs the importance placed on a patient's right to privacy.

Health Insurance Portability and Accountability Act

The Health Insurance Portability and Accountability Act (HIPAA) is a Federal statute that regulates the manner in which patient information is maintained, used, and disclosed (U.S. Department of Health and Human Services, 2003). The aspect of HIPAA that addresses the privacy of health care information is known as the *privacy rule*. Section 160.102(3) states that the privacy rule applies to practitioners who transmit health information in electronic form (including fax) in connection with a transaction; the rule applies to all of a covered practitioner's health-related information, not just that transmitted electronically (Behnke, Perlin, & Bernstein, 2003).

The regulated health information is referred to as *protected health information*. HIPAA grants patients access to their protected health information, with the exception of psychotherapy notes; however, the definition of psychotherapy notes excludes the results of clinical tests and any summary of the patient's symptoms, diagnosis, functional status, treatment plan, or prognosis. Thus, HIPAA does not prevent patients from having access to much of the information contained in diagnostic reports. "At times HIPAA will preempt state law and at other times state law will preempt HIPAA" (Behnke, Perlin, & Bernstein, 2003, p. 164). The clinician must comply with the law that affords the patient greatest access to health information and greatest privacy from third parties.

Forensic Considerations

When an individual places her mental state at issue in a legal matter, certain rights are waived in the interest of justice, including the right to privacy of relevant information. Discovery requirements allow the defense (in civil litigation) access to all relevant information upon which expert opinions are based. In forensic evaluation contexts, HIPAA constraints are limited (Connell & Koocher, 2003; Fisher, 2003). HIPAA states that information compiled in anticipation of use in *civil, criminal, and administrative* proceedings is not subject to the same right of review and amendment as is health care information in general [§164.524(a)(1)(ii)] (U.S. Department of Health and Human Services, 2003). In addition, HIPAA's privacy rule allows covered practitioners to disclose protected health information in response to a court order (§164.524), but such disclosure should be limited to the information explicitly covered by the order.

In many forensic contexts, the person being evaluated is not "the client." That is, the mental health professional is retained by a third party, such as an attorney. In such contexts, the clinician–patient relationship differs in important ways from that of clinical contexts (Bush, Barth, Pliskin, et al., 2005), including control over the release of confidential information. The mental health professional must clarify with all parties from the outset the nature of confidentiality and the manner in which information and data obtained during the evaluation will be protected and released.

Once a determination has been made that patient communications must be disclosed, it is important to determine which information will be shared and the manner in which the information will be disclosed. In making these determinations, two principles should be considered, the *Parsimony Principle* and the *Law of No Surprises* (Behnke, Perlin, & Bernstein, 2003).

The Parsimony Principle indicates that only the information necessary to achieve the purpose of the disclosure should be released. The Law of No Surprises indicates that all reasonable steps should be taken to inform patients at the outset of the relationship of the circumstances under which disclosure of information to a third party will occur. This principle "is founded upon a clinical truism: You never want your client to be surprised when you disclose confidential information ... disclosure of information should be done together with the client whenever possible" (Behnke, Perlin, & Bernstein, 2003, p. 30). Clinicians may need to educate those who are involved in the patient's life but have not been authorized to receive patient information about confidentiality requirements. In addition, it may be important to discuss confidentiality issues with the patient in private.

The freedom of competent adults to allow or restrict access to their bodies, thoughts, and feelings has long been a fundamental value of medicine and the cornerstone of mental health treatment, and clinicians are obligated to defend that value. With solid training and a personal commitment to patient welfare, geriatric mental health professionals are well positioned to do so.

INFORMED CONSENT

The right to be fully informed regarding proposed mental health services and to consent to, or decline, participation as a result of that information is based on the principle of *autonomy*. In general, clinicians inform patients of the anticipated parameters of the proposed services, including the nature and purpose of the services, fees, involvement of third parties, potential risks, and limits of confidentiality, and provide an opportunity for questions and answers.

Informing patients of the extent and limits of confidentiality should occur at the beginning of the professional relationship during the informed consent process and thereafter as needed to ensure the patient's continued understanding of her privacy rights and the exceptions to such rights. Thus, "informed consent" is not simply a form to be completed; it is an interactive *process* between the clinician and the patient that involves providing information in formats (often oral and written) that are appropriate for the patient and ensuring that the patient understands and agrees to the parameters of the proposed services; it is a process that may need to be revisited periodically as the clinical situation warrants. Although it is impossible to anticipate all of the potential threats to confidentiality, a personal commitment to ethical practice and a proactive approach to identifying and resolving ethical challenges will maximize the likelihood that the values deemed important by the patient, the clinician, and the mental health professions will find a point of mutual acceptance and satisfaction.

For patients with questionable capacity to provide consent or for those mandated for services, information about the nature and purpose of the proposed services should still be provided, and it is generally respectful and clinically helpful to seek the patient's assent. Presenting the limitations on confidentiality and the implications of failing to participate may be of particular value to the patient. With individuals who have been deemed incompetent to make medical decisions, including consenting to mental health services, and for whom a surrogate decision-maker has been appointed, the surrogate decision-maker should be fully informed and determine whether to proceed with the services. At all times, the clinician should keep the rights and welfare of the patient at the forefront of professional decision making. The consent-assent process, whether written or oral, should be documented.

Determining How Much Information to Disclose

The extent to which the potential implications of some services are conveyed to the patient must be carefully considered. Binder and Thompson (1995) observed that some patients "would choose not to undergo a neuropsychological examination if they fully understood that an abnormal result could jeopardize their normal prerogatives to make important decisions" (p. 39). For example, when a cognitive evaluation is performed to determine a patient's capacity to manage medications, pay bills, or engage in other instrumental activities of daily living, informing the patient that the results may be used as grounds for removal from the home or cessation of driving may limit the extent to which the patient agrees to participate with the evaluation.

In addition to possible refusal to participate, achievement of informed consent may interfere with the validity of the test results. Some patients may be less disclosing about psychosocial variables, premorbid history, and perceived deficits when made aware of the potential ramifications of their participation (Fisher, Johnson-Greene, & Barth, 2002). Similarly, the possibility that test results may lead to reduced independence may heighten the patient's anxiety to such an extent that it artificially deflates the test scores. Providing less specific information about the purpose of the evaluation may increase both the chances of participation and the likelihood of valid results, which may ultimately promote the health and safety of the patient, consistent with the principle of beneficence. Geriatric mental health professionals should prepare to face and work through difficult ethical challenges that pit beneficence against autonomy (American Psychological Association, 2004). To the extent possible, it is important to balance protection of older adults' safety and well-being with the right to make the decisions that govern the direction of their lives.

Clinician Values

Although the clinician's personal values cannot, and perhaps should not, be removed entirely from ethically challenging situations, the ability to identify one's own values and to separate them from the values of the patient may be necessary to promote the patient's autonomy. In some cases, preserving a patient's independence may be worth accepting some level of substandard living or some risk of patient self-injury (Norris, Molinari, & Ogland-Hand, 2002). The issues may become more complex when (a) cognitive capacity is variable or uncertain; (b) selection or appointment of the substitute decision maker is unresolved, or the surrogate appears to be pursuing an agenda that is inconsistent with the best interests of the patient; (c) pressure from multiple involved parties, such as family members, legal representatives or authorities, and institutions, conflict; and/or (d) the issues involve death and dying. In such situations, it may be natural, and perhaps necessary, for the clinician to assume a more paternalistic stance, consistent with medical tradition.

Paternalism reflects a protective, beneficent position that overrides the preferences of another (Beauchamp & Childress, 2001). As such, paternalism represents a conflict between beneficence and autonomy. Considerable caution should be exercised whenever a clinician considers, based upon her own values or beliefs, interfering with a patient's right to hold views, make choices, and take actions. As noted by Macciocchi and Stringer (2002), constraints on autonomy due to beneficence must be supported by strong clinical evidence rather than conjecture. That is, a paternalistic stance should be considered only when evidence of incapacity is clear and convincing.

It is important for the treating clinician to access colleagues and other available resources to help clarify the relevant issues, provide an uninvolved perspective, and offer assistance with choosing a course of action. To the extent that these concerns arise in the context of health care teams, families, or other systems, mental health professionals may be particularly well-suited to apply their knowledge and skills in a manner that serves to educate and facilitate communication among all parties.

When family members or others are closely involved in the life, care, or decision making of the older adult patient, everyone should be clear about the role of the clinician, who the patient is, the probable uses of information obtained, and the nature of confidentiality. It is not uncommon for family members who provide transportation and pay for services to expect to be informed of examination findings and treatment progress. However, the patient with capacity to make such decisions may ask that unfavorable results or sensitive information be withheld from family members. Careful discussion and clarification with all involved parties at the outset of the services may help avoid uncertainty and conflict.

For consent to be informed, both verbal review of consent issues and the forms reflecting consent-related information, including that related to HIPAA, must be tailored to the context in which services are provided. Because of the need to consider and prioritize state and Federal laws, ethics codes, and other resources, clinicians may be well served by consulting legal counsel when adopting procedures and forms for informed consent and other practice-related issues.

Reconciling Patient and Surrogate Values

Surrogate decision making is necessary for patients with compromised decision-making capacity. However, ethical, legal, and professional challenges emerge frequently in the context of surrogate decision making, particularly when decisions involve initiating, maintaining, or discontinuing life-sustaining procedures.

Under optimal conditions, the decisions made for patients with severe cognitive impairment are based on the known values of the patients, as documented prior to injury or illness, such as through a living will. However, as noted by Cervo, Bryan, and Farber (2006), "Despite their importance, advance directives are not a panacea because they are often overruled by surrogates, thus compromising the ethical principle of autonomy" (p. 33). Yet, when advance directives are lacking, medical decisions may be even more likely to represent the values of the surrogate decision makers, often family members, rather than the patients.

The order of which family members have preferential decision-making rights is typically established by statutory law. Frequently, the priority order begins with a legally appointed guardian, if one exists. In the absence of a legal guardian, the older adult's spouse is afforded the right to make decisions when a court has deemed the patient legally incompetent to do so. In the absence of a spouse who is able and willing to make such decisions, the decision-making authority may go to an adult child, a sibling, parents, or other nearest living relative, as specified by jurisdictional law (High, 1994).

When the values of surrogates and patients are congruent, the patients' wishes are fulfilled. However, when the values of surrogates and patients diverge, the decisions made about life-sustaining measures may not reflect the patients' values and wishes. For incompetent patients who lack clear documentation of their pre-decline values and wishes, mental health providers have an ethical obligation to strive to determine such values.

Similar to obtaining a medical and psychiatric history, obtaining a history of patients' values is often important for appropriate decision making (Doukas & McCullough, 1988). Ideally, identification and documentation of a person's basic life values and quality-of-life values is completed before significant cognitive compromise is experienced. In the absence of a documented premorbid values history, it is necessary to determine the patient's values retrospectively, with the assistance of another who knew the patient well prior to the onset of the neurological injury or illness. It is recommended that descriptions of the patient's values be obtained from at least two persons who knew the patient well prior to the cognitive decline. If discrepancies in their opinions exist, additional opinions should be sought from others.

In addition to describing the patient's values, it is recommended that surrogate decision makers provide information regarding their own values, so that the values of the patient and surrogate can be compared (see Appendix B). At times, because of their emotional involvement with the patient or other motivations, surrogates may be tempted to make decisions that are contrary to the wishes previously conveyed by the patient. The process of examining their own values can help surrogates identify when their decisions represent their values rather than the patient's values, so that they can modify their decisions appropriately. Thus, obtaining values histories for patients *and* their surrogates can be beneficial for carrying out patients' wishes. Of course, surrogates who intentionally violate the wishes of the patients will not benefit from such review.

Because of the often complex and emotionally charged nature of the decisions being made, surrogates, whether legally appointed and authorized or not, may not understand the true nature of patient's illness or condition; as a result, they often turn to physicians and other professionals for education, guidance, and assistance with making life-altering decisions (Cervo, Bryan, & Farber, 2006; High, 1994). In such instances, clinicians have a moral and ethical obligation to consider the best interests of the patient and to try to limit the impact on their decisions of nonclinical factors, such as nursing homes being reimbursed at a higher rate for residents with feeding tubes than residents who eat independently or are hand-fed (Cervo et al., 2006).

Learning Exercises

1. Define privacy, confidentiality, and privilege.
2. Describe the relationship between general bioethical principles and informed consent.
3. Describe how you can determine if a surrogate decision maker is basing health care decisions on her values or on the values of the compromised person.

9 Assessment

Dr. B, a neuropsychologist in a rural hospital, is asked to assess the cognitive status of a 79-year-old man who recently became ventilator-dependent secondary to advanced chronic obstructive pulmonary disease. A review of medical records reveals that the patient lived alone but received considerable assistance from his daughter prior to his hospitalization. The results of the neuropsychological evaluation will have direct implications for discharge planning. During a clinical interview, the patient appears depressed and moderately confused, with his involvement in the interview limited by fatigue and difficulty speaking due to his tracheostomy tube. Attempts to have the patient communicate through writing are minimally successful because the patient frequently becomes frustrated and appears to lose his train of thought. Despite attempts to inform the patient about the nature and purpose of the evaluation, Dr. B is uncertain if the patient fully understands the particulars of the evaluation. Nonetheless, after the patient's attending physician enters the room and reassures the patient that he needs to participate in the evaluation, the patient agrees to undergo the testing.

IDENTIFY THE PROBLEM

Despite the patient's apparent agreement to participate, Dr. B remains unsure about whether it is appropriate to proceed. Dr. B is concerned both about the patient's level of understanding of the evaluation process and the ability to administer tests to this patient in the manner in which they were standardized. For example, tests of spatial skills are typically completed with the dominant hand, which is how the tests are standardized. Similarly, many tests require a verbal response. Although test administration can be modified for patients who cannot use their dominant hand or cannot provide verbal responses, the potential effects of such modifications on the validity of test data are largely unknown.

Thus, Dr. B is faced with questions related to informed consent and the appropriate use of assessment instruments. Specifically, Dr. B wonders whether the patient possesses an appropriate understanding of the particulars of the evaluation to make an informed decision regarding his desire to participate. Dr. B considers whether to contact the patient's daughter for permission to proceed with testing. Finally, Dr. B considers whether the patient's need for special accommodations will result in inappropriate use of the assessment measures.

CONSIDER THE SIGNIFICANCE OF THE CONTEXT AND SETTING

Working in an inpatient medical setting that generally has short lengths of stay, Dr. B understands the need to complete evaluations as soon as possible. However, in reviewing this case, Dr. B recognizes that no extenuating circumstances, such as decisions about surgery, require immediate completion of the evaluation. In contrast, extenuating circumstances may necessitate delaying the evaluation. Dr. B understands that the multidisciplinary treatment approach employed by the hospital means that several colleagues are available who can offer preliminary insight into the patient's cognitive status and communication ability, which may be satisfactory until an appropriate neuropsychological evaluation can be performed. However, in this rural setting, he has no other local neuropsychology colleagues with which to consult.

DETERMINE PATIENT AND FAMILY/CAREGIVER ASSETS AND LIMITATIONS

The patient has a supportive daughter who provided considerable assistance prior to his recent decline and remains very involved in his treatment. However, now that his functioning is severely compromised, a higher level of care will be needed. His daughter's support and involvement in his care will remain one of the patient's primary assets.

CONSIDER OBLIGATIONS OWED

Dr. B has obligations to the patient and the referring physician and treatment team to provide information that may be of value in the patient's treatment and care, although he has a perhaps higher obligation to not conduct an inappropriate evaluation and base clinical decisions on invalid data. Dr. B also has an obligation to exchange information with the patient's daughter, who has been serving as the patient's health care proxy since his hospital admission. Dr. B also has an obligation to represent the hospital in a professional and ethical manner.

IDENTIFY AND UTILIZE RESOURCES

Dr. B reviews the relevant sections of the American Psychological Association's (2002a) Ethics Code and the Standards for Educational and Psychological Testing (SEPT; American Educational Research Association, American Psychological Association, National Council on Measurement in Education, 1999), and he consults via telephone and e-mail with a colleague who has experience working with geriatric patients in a medical setting. Through these avenues, Dr. B is able to clarify the relevant professional and ethical issues. He realizes that his primary responsibility is to ensure that his actions do not result in inappropriate decisions or treatment recommendations for the patient; instead, the evaluation should ultimately facilitate treatment and promote the patient's welfare (American Psychological Association, 2002a, General Principle A, Beneficence and Nonmaleficence).

Dr. B also understands that, to the extent possible, the patient should be involved in making the decisions that govern his medical procedures and care and his discharge (American Psychological Association, 2002a, General Principle E, Respect for People's Rights and Dignity; Standards 3.10, Informed Consent, and 9.03, Informed Consent in Assessments; SEPT Standard 8.4). However, because of the patient's deficits, the extent of his understanding of the information provided by Dr. B and other treatment team members is unknown.

Dr. B is also aware that standard administration of the test battery typically utilized on the unit will not be possible with this patient, yet any adaptations made will not be supported by research (American Psychological Association, 2002a, Standard 9.02, Use of Assessments; SEPT Standards 10.2, 10.10, and 10.11). Nevertheless, he believes that clinically valuable information can be gained by selecting and adapting tests to accommodate this patient.

CONSIDER PERSONAL BELIEFS AND VALUES

Dr. B reflects on the value that he places on autonomy. In addition, he has considerable appreciation of the dictum, "First, do no harm." Dr. B would much rather conduct no evaluation and provide no treatment recommendations to the team than perform an inappropriate evaluation and draw inaccurate conclusions or make recommendations that are inconsistent with the best interests of the patient. Determining how to optimize autonomy, do no harm, and assist the patient remains the challenge.

DEVELOP POSSIBLE SOLUTIONS TO THE PROBLEM

Concerned that the patient did not make an informed decision regarding his desire to participate in the evaluation and that the patient's expressive language difficulties would invalidate his assessment findings, Dr. B considered the following courses of action: (1) Continue with the evaluation as scheduled; (2) meet with relevant treatment team members and the patient's daughter to gain insight into the patient's functioning and to obtain assistance with determining the patient's desire to participate in the evaluation; and (3) refuse to conduct the evaluation at this time.

CONSIDER THE POTENTIAL CONSEQUENCES OF VARIOUS SOLUTIONS

1. Continuing with the evaluation may result in Dr. B's ability to answer important referral questions, or it may result in the collection of invalid data and the generation of inappropriate conclusions.
2. Obtaining additional information from the treatment team and the patient's daughter may facilitate neuropsychological decision making, or it may result in the collection of multiple subjective opinions that are of little value after a period of unnecessary delay.
3. Refusing to conduct the evaluation may result in Dr. B not taking action that is potentially harmful, but the absence of the neuropsychological evaluation may result in other team members making decisions about the patient's care that are not fully informed and thus may run counter to the patient's wishes or interests.

CHOOSE AND IMPLEMENT A COURSE OF ACTION

Having reviewed the relevant written resources and spoken with a colleague, Dr. B chose to delay the evaluation in order to consult with team members and call the patient's daughter. The attending physician agreed with the plan. The patient's speech and respiratory therapists reported that the patient appeared depressed, with variable cognition and willingness to participate in treatment. However, they indicated that the patient was less fatigued and better able to tolerate his speaking valve in the mornings. Dr. B was unable to reach the patient's daughter.

The following morning, Dr. B met with the patient, explained the purpose and nature of the evaluation, and sought the patient's assent to undergo the evaluation. The patient appeared more alert and relaxed, and appeared to agree to undergo the evaluation, although the extent of the patient's understanding of the potential implications of the evaluation remained undetermined.

Dr. B was of the opinion that failure to modify test administration to meet this patient's needs, despite a lack of research to support such modifications, would be less harmful than administering the tests in the manner in which they were standardized and interpreting the results according to norms that were based on very different populations. As a result, test administration was modified.

Test results suggested that the patient was experiencing memory and receptive language difficulties and moderate depression. Following completion of his evaluation, Dr. B was careful to report the manner in which test administration was modified and the limitations of the test results, interpretation, and recommendations.

ASSESS THE OUTCOME AND IMPLEMENT CHANGES AS NEEDED

Dr. B completed the assessment and contributed useful information to the treatment team. Plans were made for serial assessments, to include integration of the findings of other team members and information from the patient's daughter.

DISCUSSION

All clinical services begin with assessment. Although assessments can take many forms, the overarching goal of understanding the status, needs, or desires of the patient is consistent. Adequate assessment allows the clinician to move forward with the provision of services and the achievement of treatment goals. Ethical requirements, professional guidelines, and jurisdictional laws provide the parameters within which appropriate assessments occur.

In the case presented in this chapter, Dr. B was challenged to determine whether the information obtained from nonstandarized test administration would be more beneficial or harmful to the patient. In making his determination, Dr. B considered multiple resources and options, and used the ethical decision-making model to arrive at a satisfactory solution.

Thorough assessment of cognitive, psychiatric, or behavioral symptoms in the elderly is preferably interdisciplinary in nature (American Psychological Association, 2004). As part of such a process, clinicians employ methods that are deemed necessary to answer the referral questions and address other issues that they may identify as clinically important. The use of standardized neuropsychological tests may represent the most important and unique contribution that neuropsychologists can make to the assessment of dementia and age-related cognitive decline (American Psychological Association Presidential Task Force on the Assessment of Age-Consistent Memory Decline and Dementia, 1998). In the selection of assessment methods, neuropsychologists strive to be familiar with the theory, research, and practice of their methods with older adults, and to select instruments that are psychometrically appropriate for this population (American Psychological Association, 2002a, Ethical Standard 9.02, Use of Assessments; American Psychological Association, 2004; Bush & Martin, 2005; SEPT Standard 12.3).

Neuropsychological tests have increasingly been developed with higher age ranges in mind, and geriatric norms have been developed for measures previously applicable only to younger adults (Heaton, Miller, Taylor, & Grant, 2004; Lucas, Ivnik, Willis, Ferman, Smith, Parfitt, et al., 2005). However, situations still arise in which assessment of geriatric patients requires modification of standardized measures or procedures or in which representative norms are unavailable (Caplan & Shechter, 2005). Neuropsychologists working with older adults develop skill in tailoring evaluations to accommodate both the specific characteristics of the patient and the context in which the evaluation is performed (American Psychological Association, 2004). Neuropsychologists working with older adults are also familiar with the problems inherent in using assessment instruments created for younger persons.

A primary concern for neuropsychologists in recent years involves the impact of managed care on the selection and use of assessment procedures. In an effort to control costs, most managed care companies have set unreasonable limits on the number of hours of testing and the specific tests that will be reimbursed. These restrictions are often made by persons who do not have the requisite education or training to determine the parameters that constitute an appropriate neuropsychological evaluation. The restrictions place undue burden on clinicians to provide services that they may otherwise consider inadequate or inappropriate. Consistent with professional ethics, clinicians must base their diagnoses, opinions, and recommendations on information and techniques sufficient to substantiate their findings (American Psychological Association, 2002a; Ethical Standard 9.01, Bases for Assessments). Clinicians must be allowed to select the assessment methods that they consider to be appropriate for a given patient based on their education, training, and experience, and on their understanding of evidence-based assessment research (Bush, in press b).

When managed care companies attempt to control the assessment methods and procedures employed by clinicians, they place clinicians in a bind: limit the assessment performed or risk not being paid for what is considered a medically necessary service. This bind may be alleviated in some contexts by informing patients of the assessment options and the restrictions placed on payment for assessment services by managed care, and providing patients with the option of paying the balance. However, regardless of payment issues, clinicians have a responsibility to perform appropriate evaluations. This approach is consistent with the position that care should be provided by clinicians, not managed by unqualified persons.

Computerized Testing

Computerized test administration is a requirement or option for many newly developed tests. However, some older adults may be less familiar and comfortable with computers than are younger patients. Before administering tests via computer, clinicians should assess the patient's level of comfort with such procedures, substitute paper-and-pencil versions of tests when possible, and describe any limits to interpretation based on the use of information technology (Browndyke, 2005; Schatz, 2005). Neuropsychologically vulnerable patients are particularly entitled to increased protection from the potential negative effects of information technology use (Bush, Naugle, & Johnson-Greene, 2002).

Response Validity Determinations

In the interpretation of assessment results, which may include computer-generated analyses, clinicians are responsible for considering the purpose of the evaluation, situational factors, and personal characteristics of the examinee that may impact the accuracy of the interpretation (American Psychological Association, 2002a, Standard 9.06, Interpreting Assessment Results). For most evaluations, an initial step in the interpretation process is making a determination regarding the validity of the information and data obtained (American Academy of Clinical Neuropsychology, 2007; Bush, Ruff, Tröster, et al., 2005). That is, the clinician must answer the question, "Did the patient approach the evaluation in an open and honest manner and put forth good effort on the cognitive tests?"

There are many reasons why the information or data obtained from the patient may not be a valid representation of the patient's true neuropsychological status. Such reasons include "sensory deficits, fatigue, medication side effects, physical illness and frailness, discomfort or disability, poor motivation, financial disincentives, depression, anxiety, not understanding the test instructions, and lack of interest" (American Psychological Association Presidential Task Force on the Assessment of Age-Consistent Memory Decline and Dementia, 1998). Additional reasons include distrust of medical professionals, opposition to the purpose of the evaluation, and unconscious reasons such as those underlying a somatoform disorder.

Within the contexts in which many geriatric evaluations are performed, malingering seems to occur relatively infrequently. However, as just listed, many other factors may also affect response validity and, if not considered, will subsequently contribute to the development of inaccurate conclusions regarding the patient's actual level of neuropsychological functioning. Thus, the assumption that symptom validity assessment is unnecessary with older adults reflects a limited appreciation of the various factors that may compromise the validity of a patient's responses and performance (Bush & Martin, 2005). Neuropsychologists in any setting or evaluation context must "attempt to assess these sources of error and to limit and control them to the extent that they are able" (American Psychological Association Presidential Task Force on the Assessment of Age-Consistent Memory Decline and Dementia, 1998).

The manner in which response validity is assessed varies depending on the context of the evaluation. Assessment of response validity may include specific tests, validity scales, empirically derived indicators embedded within neurocognitive tests, observations, comparisons, and/or other procedures. Determination of how to assess response validity is determined by the clinician, given the unique context of the evaluation and the characteristics of the patient.

Learning Exercise

1. Standardized testing of memory and other cognitive abilities is an important aspect of the evaluations of many older adults. However, sensory and motor problems, which are more common with older adults than younger adults, may co-exist with memory deficits and interfere with standard administration of cognitive tests. How should such situations be managed?

10 Treatment

Dr. D, a psychiatrist, has provided services to a 67-year-old Filipino woman twice in 4 weeks in an inner-city outpatient geriatric mental health clinic. The patient was referred for mental health treatment by her primary medical doctor because her nearly continuous coughing, which began 3 months prior following the death of her oldest child, seemed to have no medical basis. Dr. D hypothesized that the coughing was a physical manifestation of depression related to the loss of the patient's adult child, and she prescribed an antidepressant medication. She also ordered individual psychotherapy with a counseling intern and group therapy with one of the clinic's social workers. However, problems emerged when the intern, who had training in gestalt therapy, questioned her supervisor about the evidence base for such therapy in this case, and some of the other patients in the group therapy refused to attend the group because of their fears of contracting a "coughing disease" from the patient. Based on a case conference about the patient, the treatment team wondered whether the pharmacologic approach should be the intervention of choice and the other therapies discontinued. However, Dr. D asked the team if such as treatment plan was in the patient's best interests or was a way of simplifying the problems that came with the patient.

IDENTIFY THE PROBLEM

Dr. D must balance what she thinks are treatments of choice for the patient with the clinic's ability to provide such treatments and the potential effects of the prescribed treatments on the clinic's other patients. With the clinic's emphasis on providing evidence-based treatment, adequate research may not exist to support gestalt therapy with this particular patient. Additionally, the loss of other patients from the group therapy because of their fear of contracting an illness from the patient raises questions about whether the potential benefit to the patient is worth the loss of the potential to benefit others.

CONSIDER THE SIGNIFICANCE OF THE CONTEXT AND SETTING

A variety of treatment opportunities exist in the clinic. However, there is also the necessity of considering the impact of one patient's treatment on the other patients receiving treatment at the clinic. Additionally, the clinic accepts patients who may not have the resources to be treated in other settings; thus, the patients may be forced to accept whatever treatments are available within the clinic, whether or not such treatments are supported by a body of scientific evidence.

DETERMINE PATIENT AND FAMILY/CAREGIVER ASSETS AND LIMITATIONS

In this case, the patient seems to have a supportive husband, but other details about her family are unknown.

CONSIDER OBLIGATIONS OWED

The psychiatrist must consider the interest of both the patient and others who receive treatment at the clinic. She must balance competing interests and make treatment decisions, in collaboration with the other clinicians, that serve everyone concerned.

IDENTIFY AND UTILIZE ETHICAL AND LEGAL RESOURCES

Dr. D reviews the Preamble to American Medical Association's Principles of Medical Ethics, which is part of the Code of Medical Ethics (American Medical Association, Council on Ethical and Judicial Affairs, 2006). With regard to obligations owed, she finds the following, "As a member of this profession, a physician must recognize responsibility to patients first and foremost, as well as to society, to other health professionals, and to self" (p. xvi). Dr. D also reviews Principles VIII and IX of the Code of Medical Ethics (American Medical Association, 2006) which state, respectively, "A physician shall, while caring for a patient, regard responsibility to the patient as paramount" and "A physician shall support access to medical care for all people."

Dr. D also consults publications from a variety of mental health disciplines, including mental health treatment with older adults in general (American Psychological Association Working Group on the Older Adult, 1998; Knight & Satre, 1999; Lichtenberg & Hartman-Stein, 1997; U.S. Department of Health and Human Services, 1999), evidence-based mental health treatment for older adults in (Bartels, 2005; Bartels, Dums, Oxman, Schneider, Areán, Alexopoulos, & Jeste, 2003; Pinquart & Soerensen, 2001; Scogin, 2007), and issues of importance in the treatment of older adult minorities (Gerontological Society of America, Task Force on Minority Issues in Gerontology, 1994; Hinrichsen, 2006; Miles, 1999).

CONSIDER PERSONAL BELIEFS AND VALUES

Dr. D believes that all of her patients deserve at least trials of various forms of treatment, confident that it is better to try something, even when a body of supportive evidence is currently lacking, than to withhold or postpone treatment until research identifies a preferred course of treatment. Additionally, her position is that the potential benefit to many people outweighs the potential benefit to one. She also understands that some patients from some cultures may be more prone to expressing emotional distress through physical symptoms than by reporting feelings associated with depression or other emotional reactions.

DEVELOP POSSIBLE SOLUTIONS TO THE PROBLEM

Dr. D considers the following options: (1) Continue the antidepressant medication and individual psychotherapy but discontinue group therapy; (2) continue the antidepressant medication but discontinue both individual and group therapy; (3) discharge the patient from the clinic and attempt to find a Filipino psychiatrist to whom the patient could be referred; or (4) continue the treatment plan as is, with the hope that the other members of the group therapy will understand that the cough "is all in the patient's head" and will not drop out of the group.

CONSIDER THE POTENTIAL CONSEQUENCES OF VARIOUS SOLUTIONS

Dr. D considers the following possible consequences for each of the potential solutions:

1. Continuing the pharmacologic and psychotherapeutic treatments offers a combination of therapeutic modalities, thereby maximizing opportunities for a successful outcome. Although a strong evidence base may not yet exist to support gestalt therapy with older adults who present with somatoform disorders, such treatment likely has little risk of significant adverse effects and, if it is the only type of psychotherapy available, may be better than no psychotherapy. Discontinuing the group therapy will meet the needs of other clinic patients and be an acceptable omission for this patient, who will receive combined treatment modalities anyway.
2. Continuing the pharmacologic treatment but discontinuing the individual and group therapies would only provide one aspect of a treatment plan that Dr. D believed should involve

both medication and psychotherapy; however, it would avoid the problem of not being able to provide evidence-based psychotherapy for this patient and would meet the needs of the other patients who are already receiving the group therapy.

3. Although attempting to find a potentially more qualified professional to provide services may be reasonable, discharging the patient from the clinic prematurely would essentially represent abandonment and would be unacceptable.
4. Continuing the current treatment plan would adversely affect a number of other patients, and may not be an essential component of the patient's treatment plan anyway.

CHOOSE AND IMPLEMENT A COURSE OF ACTION

Dr. D chose to pursue the first option, continuing the antidepressant medication and the psychotherapy. She spoke to the intern and his supervisor about the unique issues in this case and the need to carefully consider therapeutic techniques and the patient's reaction to psychotherapy. They agreed to meet more frequently than usual to discuss the patient's status and response to treatment. They also decided to search for a Filipino mental health professional with whom they could consult about the patient.

ASSESS THE OUTCOME AND IMPLEMENT CHANGES AS NEEDED

The patient took the antidepressant medication as prescribed and participated in the psychotherapy. After 4 weeks with essentially no change in her status, she stopped attending the psychotherapy sessions. She continued following up with Dr. D for another 3 months, still without improvement, at which point she proposed that her primary medical doctor prescribe the medication. After speaking to the primary medical doctor, Dr. D agreed with the patient's proposal and discharged her from the clinic.

DISCUSSION

Older adults respond to psychotherapy to a degree similar to younger patients, and they benefit from a variety of forms of psychological treatment (American Psychological Association, 2004). "The contextual, cohort-specific, maturity-specific challenge model provides an image of the older adult client as a mature human being facing specific problems in a given societal and familial context and with the values and views of an earlier born cohort. The specific problems, rather than the client's age, determine the techniques and goals of psychotherapy" (Knight, 2004, p. 256).

No single modality of therapy has emerged as preferable with older adults. Clinicians may adapt traditional treatments or provide therapies that have been developed specifically for use with older adults, such as reminiscence therapy. What seems clear is the importance of possessing specialized skills in treating older adults (Pinquart & Soerensen, 2001). The cohort comprised of today's older adults may have less familiarity with mental health services or may harbor more negative beliefs or feelings about mental health issues compared to subsequent cohorts (American Psychological Association, 2004). Clinicians working with the elderly must be sensitive to the potential for such attitudes to impact the working relationship or receptivity to mental health services in general and take extra care to educate the patient about the services proposed and their implications. Interestingly, when older adults are educated about potential treatments for depression, including psychopharmacologic and psychotherapeutic approaches, they tend to prefer psychologically based treatments (Scogin, 2003).

Clinicians are increasingly encouraged to provide treatments that are empirically based, and many clinicians have embraced this evolution of mental health practice. However, concern may arise that the pendulum is swinging too far in the direction of empiricism, to the extent that mental health professionals increasingly do not feel justified taking into account the subjective experience and unique needs of individual patients. Because of the emphasis on therapeutic approaches based on empirical research and the generally highly structured or specific approaches that seem to meet empirical criteria, some clinicians feel less comfortable striving to address individual needs with an empathic, integrative approach that relies more or less on different therapeutic techniques as the clinical context may warrant.

Although it is hard to argue that the efficacy of mental health treatments does not need to be established empirically, it may be equally difficult to argue that an empirically based "cookie cutter" approach to mental health treatment is appropriate for all patients. Additionally, there simply may not yet be sufficient research with various patient populations and treatment modalities to make statements about efficacy with a reasonable degree of confidence. Consistent with the bioethical principles of beneficence and nonmaleficence, and the need to respect individual differences, mental health professionals have an ethical and professional responsibility to carefully consider which treatment modality or combination of modalities is most appropriate for a given patient, based on empirical evidence to the extent possible, and then provide such treatment or make an appropriate referral.

Depending on the patient and the context, a primary goal of psychotherapy at this stage of the life cycle may be continued psychological growth. However, because many of the disorders of late adulthood are recurrent or chronic, the clinical objectives may consist of symptom management and maximization of function (Knight & Satre, 1999). Mental health professionals have an ethical obligation to facilitate patient understanding of the goals of treatment and to manage expectations appropriately. Balancing the potential benefits of maintaining hope for progress in an individual patient or family facing an unfavorable prognosis or confronting significant losses can be a particularly challenging moral and professional endeavor for clinicians.

Depression is one of the most common psychiatric disorders experienced by the elderly, and it is associated with suicide (Lebowitz, Pearson, Schneider, Reynolds 3rd, Alexopoulos, Bruce, et al., 1997; Scogin, 2003). Older adults, and men in particular, have the highest rates of suicide of any age group. Clinicians who treat older adult patients who are considering suicide, including assisted suicide, should be aware of the complex moral, ethical, professional, and legal issues involved and the resources available to guide clinicians in what may be the most professionally and emotionally trying experiences (American Psychological Association, 2003; American Psychological Association

Working Group on Assisted Suicide and End-of-Life Decisions, 2000). The American Psychological Association Working Group on Assisted Suicide and End-of-Life Decisions (2000) reported the following:

> Sweeping advances in public health, biomedical sciences, and clinical medicine ... may significantly extend life but may also confront dying individuals, their families, and health care providers with a prolonged period of dying that involves complex choices about end-of life care. These changes have resulted in the need to address end-of-life decision-making from many perspectives including medical, legal, ethical, moral, spiritual, economic, and psychosocial dimensions. There is likely to be an increasingly sophisticated demand for psychosocial services in dealing with end-of-life decisions. Furthermore, the specific issue of assisted suicide promises to become one of the most contentious and difficult social issues of our time.... In a diverse society with a variety of social and cultural values as well as a history of unequal access to medical care, issues surrounding dying and death become more complicated than in more homogeneous societies. Those working with dying persons and their families must be aware of the enormous inequities in access to and quality of health care and of the influence of profound differences in beliefs, values, and self concepts of disenfranchised people on end-of-life decision-making.

In the present case, although the patient is not facing her own death and is not considering suicide, depression manifesting as a somatoform disorder seems to be a primary cause of her persistent coughing and seems to be associated with the death of her oldest child. She is in need of a culturally appropriate approach to treatment that addresses bereavement issues and the apparent somatoform presentation and that is, to the extent possible, supported by empirical evidence. The likelihood of a parent experiencing the death of a child increases as time goes by. Therefore, older adults are more likely to have experienced the death of a child than are younger parents. The manner in which the distress associated with such losses is experienced may vary according to cultural experiences and expectations, and the appropriateness of various treatment options must take the patient's culture into account.

Learning Exercises

1.   As stated in the Preamble to American Medical Association's Principles of Medical Ethics, the doctor's/clinician's *primary* responsibility is to which of the following?

a. Patients
b. Society
c. Other health professionals
d. Self

2.   Which of the following groups has the highest rate of suicide?

a. Teenage girls
b. Older adult women
c. Middle age men
d. Older adult men

3.   Which of the following psychotherapeutic treatment modalities is preferable for older adults?

a. Psychodynamic
b. Reminiscence
c. Cognitive-behavioral
d. None of the above. Experience treating older adults supersedes any single treatment modality.

11 | Serving Special Populations

CASE 7

An 84-year-old, widowed, African American man presents to a licensed mental health counselor's office for treatment of anxiety and what his daughter describes as paranoia. The counselor, Mr. E, quickly notes that the patient is blind. He is informed that the blindness resulted from many of years of mismanagement of the patient's diabetes, which is reportedly better controlled now. The patient is also rather hard of hearing and has peripheral vascular disease. In Mr. E's estimation, the patient's anxiety and suspiciousness are the direct result of his sensory losses; that is, Mr. E believes that the patient's mind is playing tricks on him by attributing unfamiliar sounds to unknown dangers. Mr. E believes that because the patient cannot see, he cannot disprove his suspicious thoughts. Mr. E determines that he can help the patient with cognitive behavioral therapy, including teaching the patient that his anxiety-provoking thoughts are irrational. The patient's daughter wonders whether the patient could benefit from a hearing aid, but she is afraid to ask Mr. E, and Mr. E does not mention it. However, she does mention the issue to a counseling student who is training with Mr. E. Although the counseling student agrees with the patient's daughter, she does not believe that she is in a position to second-guess her supervisor. However, after observing 2 months of counseling, with essentially no benefit, the student trainee reconsiders addressing the issue with Mr. E.

IDENTIFY THE PROBLEM

Mr. E may have accurately assessed the patient's problems, but he does not seem to have considered some reasonable interventions; specifically, he did not consider the most obvious and perhaps most easily remedied intervention—recommending that the patient get a hearing aid. Despite being an otherwise competent, sensitive, and effective counselor, Mr. E does not seem to have familiarity working with older adults or persons with sensory deficits. Additionally, he does not seem to have fostered an atmosphere of open communication in his role as a supervisor of student trainees.

CONSIDER THE SIGNIFICANCE OF THE CONTEXT AND SETTING

Mr. E's private practice setting does not allow for the same ease of collaboration with colleagues found in many institutional and group practice settings. The opportunity to briefly discuss the patient's case with a colleague might have resulted in the quick identification of a hearing aid as part of the solution to the patient's problems. Similarly, the independent practice setting does not readily provide opportunities for the patient's daughter or the student trainee to discuss their ideas and concerns with other professionals.

DETERMINE PATIENT AND FAMILY/CAREGIVER ASSETS AND LIMITATIONS

The patient has a daughter who is closely involved in his life and health care and is supportive. However, she is somewhat reticent about voicing her questions and opinions to Mr. E. Issues related to gender, race, cultural background, education level, socioeconomic status, and/or other individual differences may contribute to her hesitancy to raise the question of a hearing aid with Mr. E and her father. Although she was more comfortable discussing the matter with the student trainee, the student was also reluctant to raise the seemingly innocuous hearing aid issue with Mr. E.

CONSIDER OBLIGATIONS OWED

Mr. E's primary obligation is to his patient. He has an obligation to accept as patients only persons with whom he has sufficient experience to provide a reasonably complete analysis of the problems and possible solutions; otherwise, he is obligated to consult with, or refer to, an appropriately experienced colleague. Mr. E also has an obligation to foster an atmosphere of openness with related parties, such as the patient's daughter and those whom he supervises. Such an atmosphere will allow Mr. E to better serve his patients. The student trainee also has a primary obligation to the patient.

IDENTIFY AND UTILIZE ETHICAL AND LEGAL RESOURCES

The American Counseling Association (ACA) (2005) Code of Ethics states, "The primary responsibility of counselors is to respect the dignity and to promote the welfare of clients" (Section 1.A.a. Primary Responsibility). When counselors have questions about their ability to serve a certain patient or patient population, including when they engage in a new practice specialty, they must refer the patient or consult with an experienced colleague (Sections C.2.a, C.2.b, and C.2.e). Developmental and cultural considerations are emphasized throughout the Code of Ethics (e.g., A.2.c. Developmental and Cultural Sensitivity). Additionally, the Code advises, "Counselors develop positive working relationships and systems of communication with colleagues to enhance services to clients" (Section D, Introduction).

Working with special populations, including older adults, diverse populations, and persons with disabilities, requires particular sensitivity to general bioethical principles of justice and respect for the autonomy and dignity of competent adults. In the role of supervisor, mental health professionals must be aware of the power differential between supervisor and supervisee and proactively facilitate reciprocal communication regarding patients and the conceptualization and application of treatment options (ACA, 2005, Section F.3.e. Potentially Beneficial Relationships). The Code of Ethics of the National Board of Certified Counselors (2005) also requires counselors to uphold the values of the profession that are described here, with a primary responsibility to respect the integrity and promote the welfare of clients (Section B.1). Student trainees have the same obligations to patients as do professional counselors (ACA, 2005, Section F.8.a. Standards for Students).

In addition to professional ethics, Federal laws address the importance of making appropriate services available to persons with disabilities, including disabilities resulting from sensory impairments and emotional disorders. Both Section 504 of the Rehabilitation Act of 1973 (see also Rehabilitation Act Amendments of 1992) and Title II of the Americans with Disabilities Act (ADA) of 1990 prohibit covered providers from discriminating against persons with disabilities in the provision of services on the basis of their disability. However, these programs apply only to programs that receive Federal financing or are conducted by public entities, such as governmental agencies. Thus, by virtue of the private practice setting, Mr. E is not considered a covered entity. However, even if he were a covered entity, his failure to consider recommending a hearing aid as part of his intervention may not reflect discrimination as defined by the Rehabilitation Act of 1973 and the ADA (see www.hhs.gov/ocr/504.html and www.ada.gov/).

The student also has access to the training director in her Master's degree program. Training directors often have prior experiences with the professionals who provide supervision to students from the program, and they are able to draw upon those experiences when advising current trainees. Thus, training directors can be excellent resources for student trainees who are concerned about challenging professional, ethical, and supervisory experiences.

CONSIDER PERSONAL BELIEFS AND VALUES

Mr. E is invested in both providing appropriate services for his patients and providing good training opportunities for his trainees, and he believes that he is accomplishing both goals in his work with the patient in this case. However, he also believes that as an educated and licensed professional, he knows better than family members or students how to identify salient problems and achieve treatment goals. As a result, he does not seek nor particularly welcome questions or concerns from others.

The student trainee believes that she has a responsibility ensure that her patients receive appropriate services and recommendations. However, she also believes that confronting Mr. E, however tactfully, could adversely affect her ability to successfully complete her training and receive a positive letter of recommendation. Thus, she considers the potentially competing demands of wanting to help the patient but not wanting to sabotage her current training and future career.

DEVELOP POSSIBLE SOLUTIONS TO THE PROBLEM

The student trainee considers the following options: (1) Discuss with Mr. E both her wish for more open communication in the supervisory relationship and the possibility of recommending that the patient pursue hearing aids, (2) discuss with Mr. E the hearing aid issue only, (3) encourage the patient's daughter to pursue hearing aids for the patient without discussing the issue with Mr. E, (4) directly recommend to the patient that he pursue hearing aids, or (5) bide her time until her training rotation with Mr. E ends.

CONSIDER THE POTENTIAL CONSEQUENCES OF VARIOUS SOLUTIONS

   1. Discussing the need for more open communication will likely directly affect the remainder of the student's training experience with Mr. E, either positively or negatively; however, it also

has a high probability of getting Mr. E to make a straightforward recommendation about hearing aids that will be of value to the patient.

2. Discussing the hearing aid issue with Mr. E only will likely achieve the desired benefit for the patient but will leave the nature of the supervisory relationship unaddressed, thereby limiting the potential richness of the experience, but also providing a "safer" option for the student trainee.

3. Encouraging the daughter to pursue the hearing aid issue would likely be of little value, because the patient's daughter has already considered the question of hearing aids and made the decision not to pursue them, although gentle encouragement from a professional (which is how she views the student trainee) may help resolve any potential ambivalence. This option, by circumventing Mr. E, may also undermine his authority and, if he finds out, negatively affect the supervisory relationship.

4. Making a direct recommendation to the patient seems reasonable but, because the student trainee is only observing therapy sessions conducted by Mr. E, such a recommendation coming from her may be perceived as undermining the therapeutic dyad.

5. Doing nothing, while posing no risk for the student trainee, is of no benefit for either the patient or the supervisory experience.

CHOOSE AND IMPLEMENT A COURSE OF ACTION

After discussing the matter with her training director, the student trainee decides to pursue the first option. During the next supervision session, she raises the issue of the hearing aids and then inquires about whether they can discuss the nature of the supervision.

ASSESS THE OUTCOME AND IMPLEMENT CHANGES AS NEEDED

Mr. E is receptive to recommendations regarding hearing aids but seems somewhat defensive about not having thought of it himself.

With regard to discussing the nature of the supervision, Mr. E agrees to do so but seems only minimally invested in the endeavor until ultimately directing his attention to other issues. However, his subsequent interactions with the student trainee do not seem to have been affected by her concerns. The student trainee continues to process these issues with her training director. The training director decides to reconsider Mr. E's practice as an appropriate training site for future students.

DISCUSSION

This case illustrates how a seemingly innocuous issue (i.e., whether to recommend pursuing hearing aids) can have numerous professional and ethical implications that must be carefully considered. It may be easy to simply wonder, "Why not just encourage the patient to get his hearing checked and consider hearing aids? What's the big deal?" However, personalities, interpersonal dynamics, power differentials, and patient and family characteristics are among the issues that must be carefully considered even in circumstances that may seem straightforward on the surface. In this case, the potential interaction of sensory deficits and psychiatric symptoms was explored, with sensory problems being overlooked in favor of psychiatric symptoms. However, the risk also exists that valid psychiatric problems can be misattributed to sensory or cognitive deficits. Mental health professionals who work with older adults must be sensitive to common physical and psychiatric comorbidities.

Ethical practice requires particular attention to the welfare of vulnerable patients. Physical frailty, cognitive or sensory impairment, cultural and linguistic diversity, disability, and other characteristics of the patient may increase vulnerability to inappropriate and potentially harmful conclusions and/or care by mental health professionals who are insensitive to the relevance and importance of such factors. In addition, a combination of these factors in a given patient increases the demand on clinicians to exercise care during both the evaluation and treatment process (Byrd & Manly, 2005; Iverson & Slick, 2003).

Personal and societal biases exist toward some groups with which geriatric mental health clinicians have professional contact, and clinicians are not immune from such biases. Clinicians must be aware of how biases regarding age, gender, ethnicity, disability, and other patient characteristics may interfere with the objective provision of mental health services, including evaluations, and strive to overcome possible biases or refer the patient to another mental health professional (American Counseling Association, 2005, C.5. Nondiscrimination; American Psychological Association, 2002b; American Psychological Association Presidential Task Force on the Assessment of Age-Consistent Memory Decline and Dementia, 1998; National Board of Certified Counselors, 2005, A12).

Ethnic, cultural, and linguistic factors are essential influences on patient behavior in medical and mental health care settings. With the exception of some purely biomedical tests, the results of evaluation and treatment services may be influenced by ethnic, cultural, and linguistic factors. However, the extremely variable experiential, attitudinal, and behavioral differences that distinguish patients between and within ethnic and cultural groups challenge clinicians to reach accurate and meaningful assessment conclusions (Brickman, Cabo, & Manly, 2006; Byrd & Manly, 2005).

Although the ethical clinician considers age, gender, race, disability, and other factors when providing services, the specific impact of these factors on the test results or therapeutic experience of any given patient can often be very difficult to discern. Questions exist regarding when or whether to evaluate persons whose cultural background differs from that of the clinician or the dominant U.S. culture (Fletcher-Janzen, Strickland, & Reynolds, 2000; Nell, 2000; Samuda, 1998; Sandoval, Frisby, Geisinger, et al., 1998). As Hinrichsen (2006) stated, "Issues of race and ethnicity figure in the lives of older adults and their service providers in ways that may not be readily apparent" (p. 29).

Additionally, racial and cultural differences often exist between older adults and their health care aides, many of whom are foreign-born, particularly in urban areas (Hinrichsen, 2006). These aides tend to be paid at the low end of the salary spectrum and often do not receive the recognition or appreciation that they deserve for their work in caring for physically, neurologically, and/or psychiatrically compromised older adults. This lack of appreciation may stem from a variety of misunderstandings about persons from different cultures or may be based in long-standing and deeply held beliefs on the part of the older adult. Older adults who receive care from persons from different racial or cultural backgrounds may worry that such aides will hold different values, not understand their needs, and/or talk about them in a language that they do not understand. However, the dignity, morale, and ultimate effectiveness of the aides can suffer as a result of older adults' misperceptions, suspiciousness, and abusive comments or actions. The work of mental health professionals in such contexts is not to challenge or attempt to change the older adult's long-held beliefs but instead to try to understand them (Hinrichsen, 2006). Thus, the clinician's efforts may need to be geared toward modifying the older adult patient's behavior, so that the aide's feelings and efforts do not suffer, and the older adult receives the care that he or she needs.

The subspecialty of ethnogeriatrics is devoted to providing education and training to assist clinicians in developing competence in working with ethnically diverse older adults (see, for example, sgec.stanford.edu/resources). Toward the development of increased professional competence at the intersection of multicultural issues and aging, Hinrichsen (2006) advised three primary steps for mental health professionals: Learn more, teach more, and talk more. Geriatric mental health professionals who work with disabled, diverse, or otherwise unique populations of older adults have a responsibility to initiate conversations with colleagues, trainees, caregivers, and others about these complex issues (Comas-Diaz & Jacobsen, 1991). Such conversation is a primary and ongoing step toward maximizing the care, treatment, and well-being of older adult patients.

In addition to providing clinical services to vulnerable populations, mental health professionals who educate or train students are, in effect, working with another vulnerable group. Despite efforts on behalf of supervisors to provide an atmosphere of openness, collaboration, and mutual respect, the student role is inevitably a position of vulnerability. Students and trainees are well aware that their words or behaviors can affect their educational or training experience and have considerable long-term effects on their careers. In such a context, there is little incentive for students or trainees to take risks, even when potentially risky actions may benefit patients. Although supervisors cannot eliminate the power differential with student trainees, all parties are well served when supervisors continually strive to provide a supportive atmosphere of open communication and invite novel ideas from trainees, including questions about the supervisors choices or actions.

Learning Exercises

1. How do cultural or disability issues affect older adult recipients of mental health services in your practice context?

2. Describe a clinical situation with which you are familiar that you believe could have been better handled if greater attention had been paid to cultural or disability issues.

3. What can you do to assure that similar situations will be handled more effectively in the future?

Health Promotion

Dr. F, a psychologist, gives a lecture at a local library about minimizing the risk of Alzheimer's disease (AD). The title of the lecture, as presented in marketing materials, is "Prevent Alzheimer's Disease: 5 Easy Daily Steps." As part of her presentation, Dr. F describes the incidence of dementia in the elderly and gives case studies of lives tragically changed by dementing disorders. This aspect of the presentation invariably gets the audience's attention and raises concerns about developing AD. She then describes the exciting emerging scientific literature on the various ways to reduce the risk of developing AD, including appropriate nutritional intake, physical activity, mental activity, stress reduction, and maintenance of overall health. The research findings give the audience hope. Dr. F then describes her practice, which includes her patent-pending "AD busting" mental exercise program. She concludes with the statement, "If you want to avoid Alzheimer's disease, start your AD busting program now. It's never too late!" After the lecture, Dr. F hands out her business cards and brochures and tells interested audience members that she accepts Medicare and private pay. A retired psychologist, Dr. G, sitting the in audience, finds the content of the lecture informative but the process rather distasteful, and she wonders about the ethical and legal implications of Dr. F's presentation and practices.

IDENTIFY THE PROBLEM

Dr. G believes that Dr. F is preying upon the fears of older adults and promoting a solution to the fears that is, at best, overstated based on the available research. Although, when presented the right way with the right expectations and cautions, there can be a very important role for mental health professionals in the promotion of neurological health, making such definitive statements about the value of an unproven product can be misleading. By triggering the fears of the audience and then offering her services as the possibly only and apparently guaranteed solution, Dr. F's approach is rather coercive. Additionally, the content of her marketing materials and her billing of Medicare for preventative services both seem to be inappropriate. Dr. G must decide how to address these issues, if at all.

CONSIDER THE SIGNIFICANCE OF THE CONTEXT AND SETTING

In the relatively informal community library setting, there is little chance of professional oversight. As a result, Dr. F is likely to get away with making strong, intimidating, and unsupportable statements, and she is likely to benefit financially in the process. In the current case, however, a retired colleague happened to be attending the lecture and may elect to address the areas of concern.

DETERMINE PATIENT AND FAMILY/CAREGIVER ASSETS AND LIMITATIONS

In this case, no specific patient exists. Dr. F's community lectures are typically attended by older adults who live and function independently, but are concerned about perceived increases in forgetfulness, family histories of dementia, or risks of dementia as presented in the news or other popular media. Thus, compared to other treatment contexts, the older adults who attend the lectures are high functioning and invested in remaining that way. However, because they are independent, there is less involvement of younger family members who may be more skeptical of Dr. F's claims.

CONSIDER OBLIGATIONS OWED

Dr. F has obligations to the public, including persons who attend her lectures. She has additional obligations to those who choose to pursue her "Alzheimer's prevention" services. She also has a legal obligation to not bill Medicare for preventative services that are typically not covered services. In addition, Dr. G, although retired, has a moral obligation to try to protect her age-related peers by addressing Dr. F's apparently inappropriate statements and behaviors.

IDENTIFY AND UTILIZE ETHICAL AND LEGAL RESOURCES

Dr. F is ethically mandated to describe her lectures in terms that are honest and do not generate undue fear or overstate the known value of her services. In Standard 5.01 (Avoidance of False or Deceptive Statements), the Ethics Code of the American Psychological Association (2002a) states the following:

> (a) Public statements include but are not limited to paid or unpaid advertising, product endorsements, grant applications, licensing applications, other credentialing applications, brochures, printed matter, directory listings, personal resumés or curricula vitae, or comments for use in media such as print or electronic transmission, statements in legal proceedings, lectures and public oral presentations, and published materials. Psychologists do not knowingly make public statements that are false, deceptive, or fraudulent concerning their research, practice, or other

work activities or those of persons or organizations with which they are affiliated.

(b) Psychologists do not make false, deceptive, or fraudulent statements concerning (1) their training, experience, or competence; (2) their academic degrees; (3) their credentials; (4) their institutional or association affiliations; (5) their services; (6) the scientific or clinical basis for, or results or degree of success of, their services; (7) their fees; or (8) their publications or research findings.

Similarly, Dr. F maintains responsibility for statements in advertising and marketing materials that have been made by others (Standard 5.03, Descriptions of Workshops and Non-Degree-Granting Educational Programs). She is also required to "not engage, directly or through agents, in uninvited in-person solicitation of business from actual or potential therapy clients/patients or other persons who because of their particular circumstances are vulnerable to undue influence" (Standard 5.06, In-Person Solicitation). The fear of developing Alzheimer's disease that Dr. F generates in audience members during the first part of her presentation may have the appearance, whether intentional or not, of being done for the purpose of making them more receptive (i.e., vulnerable) to her proposed services. Although "community outreach services" are listed as an exception in Standard 5.06, the underlying bioethical principle of respecting patient autonomy may be threatened when strong emotional reactions (e.g., fear of developing AD) are elicited in a context that funnels people into one's own professional practice with the promise of a solution that has yet to be substantiated.

The Ethics Code of the American Psychological Association (2002a), which governs Dr. F's professional behavior, further states the following:

(b) When obtaining informed consent for treatment for which generally recognized techniques and procedures have not been established, psychologists inform their clients/patients of the developing nature of the treatment, the potential risks involved, alternative treatments that may be available, and the voluntary nature of their participation. (Standard 10.01, Informed Consent to Therapy)

Thus, Dr. F has a responsibility to establish reasonable expectations regarding the potential value of her services and to not overstate the established effectiveness of the strategies and techniques that she provides or for which she advocates.

Dr. G, although retired and no longer subject to the ethics code that previously governed her approach to ethical conflict resolutions, recalls the appropriate steps to take when attempting to resolve perceived ethical violations by colleagues. Specifically, she knows that an informal resolution is preferred in many situations (Standard 1.04, Informal Resolution of Ethical Violations). Therefore, she considers bringing her concerns to Dr. F's attention. She also intends to raise the issue of possible fraudulent billing of Medicare. Although the False Claims Act (1986; also known as the "Lincoln Law"[1]) reinforces "whistle blowing" by providing the person who reports the fraudulent act with a portion (typically 15%–25%) of recovered damages, Dr. G is not motivated by a possible monetary reward; she simply believes she has a responsibility to address the potential problem.

Dr. G also considers contacting colleagues or an ethics committee for other perspectives. However, she believes that the American Psychological Association's (2002a) Ethics Code was clear, and she understands the issues well enough to make an informed decision about how to address the problem.

CONSIDER PERSONAL BELIEFS AND VALUES

Dr. G wants to believe that Dr. F is not intentionally trying to prey upon the fears of older adults for her personal financial gain. She leans toward the possibility that Dr. F is concerned about the significant public health concerns involving AD and is trying to educate the public and offer solutions that promote both brain health and hope. However,

---

[1] The Federal Claims Act was originally passed 1863, and was amended in 1943 and 1986. Several states have enacted similar statutes with *qui tam* provisions that allow a private individual who assists in a prosecution to receive part of the financial penalty. See also *United States ex rel. Friedrich LU v. David W. OU, et al.* (2004) and *Vermont Agency of Natural Resources v. United States ex rel. Stevens* (2000).

Dr. G realizes that, regardless of Dr. F's motivations, her own value of protecting others, and vulnerable populations in particular, require that she address the matter.

DEVELOP POSSIBLE SOLUTIONS TO THE PROBLEM

Dr. G realizes that her options consist of avoiding or addressing the matter. Because of her value system, Dr. G knows that avoiding the problem is not an acceptable option. Once she is committed to addressing the problem, she considers whether her action should be an attempt at informal resolution or a formal complaint to an ethics committee and/or Medicare.

CONSIDER THE POTENTIAL CONSEQUENCES OF VARIOUS SOLUTIONS

Dr. G understands that attempting to informally resolve most perceived ethical violations is the preferred course of action. Although confronting colleagues about ethical misconduct can be extremely awkward and uncomfortable, this option may achieve the desired results and allows for minimal damage to Dr. F's practice or reputation. Additionally, if the informal contact does not achieve the desired result, more formal steps can still be taken afterward. In contrast to the informal approach, making formal complaints will likely achieve the desired result but may occur at significant and unnecessary emotional, financial, and professional costs to Dr. F.

CHOOSE AND IMPLEMENT A COURSE OF ACTION

Dr. G elects to pursue an informal resolution of the problem. After the presentation, she takes Dr. F's business card. A few days later, she calls Dr. F, introduces herself as a retired psychologist, and presents her concerns. Dr. F is defensive and states that she is just presenting the state of the science as it currently exists. She adamantly denies trying to instill or increase fear in the attendees, and she takes the position that she would be negligent to not offer solutions to the problem, including her practice which is the only one in the area proactively addressing memory wellness. She also denies that she is establishing unrealistic expectations regarding the value of her memory exercise program in preventing AD.

With regard to billing Medicare, Dr. F states that she performs neurocognitive testing of all interested persons prior to beginning the memory exercise program, and she only bills Medicare for the memory exercise program when testing has revealed deficits that warrant some type of diagnosis. Thus, she states that she is providing cognitive treatment in those cases, which is covered by Medicare. When asked by Dr. G, Dr. F does not acknowledge that she gives attendees the impression that everyone's memory exercise program can be covered by Medicare.

ASSESS THE OUTCOME AND IMPLEMENT CHANGES AS NEEDED

Dr. G considers the attempted informal resolution to be unsuccessful and is disappointed that she must now take additional, more formal, steps to address the problem. She contacts the ethics committee of the state psychological association, which reviews and adjudicates complaints against its members. She files a formal complaint with the ethics committee. There is no additional correspondence, and she notices over the following few months that Dr. F does not seem to be giving her community lectures. However, about a year later, she reads in a local newspaper, "Prevent Alzheimer's Disease: 5 Easy Daily Steps." She contacts the ethics committee to find out the results of their investigation. She is told that Dr. F had provided reasonable justification of her actions, and that their investigation did not reveal sufficient evidence to pursue the matter further; the case was closed. Dr. G considers whether to pursue the matter further by reporting Dr. F to another ethics committee, the state licensing board, or Medicare, but she is discouraged by the outcome of her initial efforts and decides to drop the issue.

DISCUSSION

Until recent years, treatments such as cognitive rehabilitation or memory training have been considered limited in their usefulness for individuals with age-related cognitive decline and dementia (American Psychological Association, 2004). Instead, treatments such as environmental restructuring and the use of compensatory memory aids and other strategies have been preferred. However, relatively recent research has provided support for the value of cognitive activity and exercise in late life (Ball et al., 2002; Hofmann, Hock, Kuhler, & Muller-Spahn, 1996; Moore, Sandman, McGrady, & Kesslak, 2001; Wilson et al., 2002). When mental health professionals consider recommending or providing treatments that are less well-established, it is particularly important to weigh the potential benefits against the potential risks and costs, and to involve the patient or the surrogate decision maker in the decision-making process (Bush & Martin, 2004a; Bush, 2006). The use of innovative treatments is consistent with ethical practice in those instances in which the potential costs and risks are minimal (nonmaleficence), the potential for benefit exists (beneficence), and expectations can be carefully managed (Bush & Martin, 2005).

Mental health professionals often help promote the health and well-being of older adults through the development of psychoeducational programs, involvement in community-based prevention programs, and advocacy within health care and political systems (American Psychological Association, 2004). Consistent with the principle of beneficence, clinicians can combine their clinical and consultation skills with familiarity with relevant research to promote the health and well-being of older adults in ways that extend well beyond the numbers that most clinicians reach in a more traditional clinical practice.

Although applying scientific advancements to promote healthier aging and possibly longer lives is considered by many to be a very positive contribution to society and the lives of individuals, underlying questions of whether and how to promote health and extend life have varied throughout history. Applying scientific advancements to promote longevity, often referred to as anti-aging medicine, has been a pursuit of investigators throughout much of modern history. From the 16th to 18th centuries, longevity efforts were based on the belief that old age was a period of worth that was to be embraced for the positive aspects of late life (Haber, 2004). In contrast, the anti-aging efforts during the 19th and early 20th centuries were based on the belief that later life was a time of compromised existence that should be feared and despised. The recent anti-aging movement shares the assumptions of a century ago, that old age is a disease that needs eradicating and that older adults constitute a considerable economic burden that drains society of critical resources that could be better utilized in other ways (Haber, 2004).

Biogerontologists argue that many current anti-aging procedures and products are essentially "snake oil," which at best do not achieve their promised goals and at worst are harmful (Binstock, 2004). They argue that anti-aging injections, special mineral waters, and other procedures and products are based on pseudoscience, which they distinguish from their own studies. However, many of those same biogerontologists are involved in longevity efforts (Binstock, 2004), and some of them have substantial commercial interests in the interventions they develop and the outcome of their research. Both the scientists who develop and study new anti-aging products and the clinicians who adopt new products and procedures for use with their clients have a responsibility to disclose conflicts of interest, risks, and unknowns, and to help consumers explore the meaning and implications of choosing to engage in anti-aging efforts.

The morality of pursuing immortality has long been questioned. To further address this question, Post (2004) presented a triadic ethical framework for understanding "prolongevity." Within this framework, natural law, equalitarian justice, and beneficence are examined in a balanced manner. Post concluded, "the goal of prolongevity through decelerated aging is ethically valid as a potential means to the beneficent amelioration of the many diseases for which old age is the major susceptibility factor" (p. B534).

With regard to the current case, Dr. G was essentially concerned that Dr. F, perhaps in a good faith attempt to help reduce the risk of AD, was selling "snake oil", and billing Medicare for it. She fulfilled what she believed to be her moral obligation to protect others by pursuing both informal and formal attempts to address her concerns; however, in some instances, the outcomes of such efforts are not considered satisfactory. Determining when to address the perceived ethical misconduct of colleagues and the lengths to which an acceptable remedy should be pursued can be among the most challenging decisions that clinicians have to make (Deidan & Bush, 2002).

Clinicians who do their due diligence with regard to the questionable behavior prior to addressing perceived misconduct tend to be well positioned to achieve an appropriate resolution; nevertheless, sometimes clinicians are left feeling dissatisfied, even though they did their due diligence and addressed the issue in a manner consistent with ethical protocol. When determining the extent to which perceived ethical misconduct should be pursued, clinicians should carefully consider their personal motivations and the reasonably anticipated risks and benefits associated with the various courses of action. When promoting a product or service from which one receives financial compensation or other direct benefit, mental health professionals can improve transparency regarding their motivations by disclosing to consumers the relationships—including financial relationships—that they have with the parties that benefit from the promotion. When a clinician's own practice benefits from the promotion of products or services that she provides, an obligation exists to clearly identify the limitations of the products or services that are being offered and to offer alternative options, if they exist, so that consumers can make informed choices.

Learning Exercises

1.   How do you determine when there is sufficient science to support an intervention?

2.   In your work with older adults, how do you approach perceptions of aging? For example, do you support the position that it is important to postpone the effects of aging as long as possible, perhaps through anti-aging techniques, or do you support the position that late life is a time of worth that should be experienced and appreciated in its natural course? Or, is there another position that you endorse, perhaps supporting the perspective of the individual patient? Explain your position.

Social Considerations

Many ethical and professional challenges stem from, or are encountered in, contexts that extend well beyond the individual patient, family, or facility. Community or societal trends or changes may challenge clinicians to modify their practices to meet the changing wishes or demands of consumers. Similarly, mental health practitioners may choose to put themselves or their patients in the public eye for what they consider to be a "greater good" or, perhaps, to satisfy their own narcissistic needs.

In this chapter, a sample of such situations is presented in the form of brief vignettes and discussion. In order to present multiple vignettes, this chapter does not follow the same format as the preceding chapters but instead presents the vignettes followed by a review of the problems. Nevertheless, readers may choose to apply the ethical decision-making model to each of these cases to achieve a deeper understanding of the issues and ways to address them.

CASE 9

A 67-year-old woman has been receiving psychiatric care for anxiety from the same psychiatrist for 3 years. Rapport is good, and she has benefited from the medications that he has prescribed. Within the past 6 months, she has experienced increased anxiety and has asked the psychiatrist about a medication that she has seen advertised on TV. She has become increasingly challenging in her questioning each time that she has brought the topic up for discussion, and the psychiatrist suspects that she may give him an ultimatum regarding prescribing the medication, or she will seek treatment elsewhere. Typically, the psychiatrist would not bend to such demands; however, she is the sixth patient in recent weeks to inquire about or demand the medication because of the television commercial. With two patients who recently demanded the medication, the psychiatrist carefully considered whether it would be appropriate for them but decided against it, in part because of what he considered to be insufficient research to support its widespread use. He did, however, offer to explore other treatment options with the patients. The patients, though, were firm in their demands, and terminated their treatment with the psychiatrist. The psychiatrist suspected that they would get the advertised anxiolytic from another provider, despite his belief that it would not be appropriate for them, and he became angry that the pharmaceutical industry was putting him in this bind and potentially putting patients at risk.

DISCUSSION

Direct marketing of drugs to the public seems to have become an accepted business strategy for pharmaceutical companies, with television commercials constantly informing us of easy ways to overcome erectile dysfunction, eliminate fears, remain active without pain, sleep soundly, lose weight, and live happy lives. Of course, they also quickly point out some of the possible adverse reactions, such as uncontrollable flatulence or the potential need to go to a local emergency room. However, the beautiful and seemingly content and satisfied actors that grace our television screens never seem to be in need of a change of undergarments or on their way to the ER. As a result, it is easy for us, as viewers of TV programs and recipients of the messages of the program sponsors such as pharmaceutical companies, to be curious about, and perhaps swayed by, the satisfied actors and the promised benefits of the products that leave them so satisfied. So, we do as they instruct; we talk to our doctors about the drugs to see if they're right for us. However, sometimes we, as consumers, desperate for relief from life's problems, determine before arriving at the doctor's office that the advertised medication is *the* medication for us. If we cannot get the medication from *our* doctor, we can certainly get it from *some* doctor.

As business persons and many mental health professionals know, the power of a strong marketing campaign cannot be overstated. People who are suffering from physical or mental health problems can be particularly vulnerable to such power. Mental health professionals and professional organizations should consider whether and how to address the impact of big business on clinical practice. The pharmaceutical industry has long sought to influence clinical decision making through more or less subtle campaigning and incentives to physicians. However, physicians, unlike vulnerable members of the public, understand the process and can make informed decisions about their willingness to be influenced by external forces. Thus, direct marketing to the public represents a relatively new, and potentially harmful, business ploy, and the mental health professions have a responsibility to take steps to protect vulnerable persons in this regard.

To complicate this issue further, the pharmaceutical industry has been quite profitable over time, and many mental health professionals undoubtedly include pharmaceutical companies in their investment portfolios. Some mental health professionals may be unaware that pharmaceutical companies are bundled with other companies in their money market accounts. Thus, many prescribing physicians, despite the direct impact on their clinical practices, are benefiting from the successful marketing campaigns of the pharmaceutical companies. Clinicians should consider whether it is hypocritical to invest in companies that engage in business practices that are antithetical to the welfare of their patients and other vulnerable persons. It may not be hypocritical to invest in a company without supporting all of its practices, particularly those that may be considered potentially harmful, such as direct marketing of drugs to the public. The clinician may even take steps to change actions or policies of the company that the clinician considers problematic; this option may actually be quite responsible and mutually beneficial.

CASE 10

Mr. Jones, a wealthy retired real estate developer, is admitted to a skilled nursing facility for long-term care. During the admission process, Mrs. Jones is informed by the social work case manager that she should pursue Medicaid for her husband and divert her husband's assets and their joint assets to herself and their children, so that they don't lose their life savings. The social worker states that she can help with the process, and she also recommends that a specific attorney who specializes in elder law be consulted. Mrs. Jones hears terms such as "spousal refusal" and "spend down" and becomes quite anxious. Mrs. Jones says, "My husband would hate accepting charity, and we've saved for a rainy day. Shouldn't we use our own money to pay for his care?" The social worker responds, "It's not charity, its taxes, and you paid more than your share over the years; you're entitled. Don't you want Mr. Jones' hard earned money to go to your children?" Mrs. Jones replies, "I suppose so" and begins the paperwork, but she has a very unsettling feeling inside when she gets home.

DISCUSSION

Mental health professionals have a responsibility in many contexts to advocate for their clients. An ethical obligation (beneficence) exists to use one's expertise to help educate clients about available resources when they are unfamiliar with the contexts in which they encounter the mental health professional. There is also an obligation in some contexts to help clients obtain the services and resources that they need and deserve. At the same time, an ethical obligation exists to consider the equitable distribution of services and resources (justice) when working with clients.

Government resources such as Medicaid exist to help people who do not have the financial resources to obtain needed services for themselves. Is it right for the social worker to encourage people who have considerable financial resources to "buck the system" by finding loopholes in Federal laws that allow them essentially to keep their own money and utilize public funding that exists to help those who have fewer resources? Is it right for the social worker to directly assist wealthy individuals with that process? Or, is it right for people who have worked hard and saved throughout their lives to not have access to the same Federal benefits as people who have not worked or saved as much? Are they being penalized at the end of their lives for working hard and saving?

Nursing home life can be a great equalizer. People who have worked all of their lives and spent frugally must spend all of their money on the same care that others receive after years of not working or of working and spending frivolously. Ultimately, in long-term care facilities the wealthy, the poor, and everyone in between tend to end up receiving the same care and having it covered with Medicare and Medicaid funds. As mental health professionals working with older adults, particularly when working in long-term care facilities, we have an obligation to consider our own values regarding these issues, as well as the impact of our values on the information and services we provide to our clients. By better understanding our own values and motivations, we are better positioned to help our clients understand their options and values and make the decisions that are right for them (respect for autonomy).

CASE 11

Dr. M, a psychiatrist, is on the board of directors of a not-for-profit foundation that raises money for research on Parkinson's disease. In his private practice, one of his older adult patients is a celebrity, having starred in many films throughout her life. Dr. M informs the board of directors that one of his patients is a famous actress, whom he can get to speak at their upcoming foundation fund-raising dinner. The board enthusiastically supports having Dr. M extend the invitation to his patient. When Dr. M invites his patient to be the keynote speaker the upcoming event, she initially appears hesitant. He then explains that the event will likely bring in large sums of money for a very important cause, which he thinks she can probably relate to. He tells her that having her speak will ensure the event's success. She reluctantly agrees.

DISCUSSION

Dr. M has the noble goal of helping to raise money for a worthy charity; however, he may also have, at some level of awareness, the goal of impressing the other board members and his patient. By telling the other board members that the celebrity is one of his patients, he will have violated the patient's confidentiality when the board members learn her identity (American Medical Association, 2006; Principle IV; Opinions 5.05, Confidentiality, and 10.01, Fundamental Elements of the Patient-Physician Relationship).

Additionally, because of the position of influence that Dr. M maintains as the patient's treating psychiatrist, the patient may be more prone to acquiesce to his request than she would if a psychiatrist who was not her treating doctor had contacted her. Thus, for any number of practical or therapy-related (e.g., transferential) reasons, the patient may be unduly influenced and exploited by Dr. M, whether or not that is his intention. Principles of Medical Ethics (American Medical Association, 2006) instruct Dr. M to "Recognize a responsibility to participate in activities contributing to the community and betterment of public health" (Principle VII), which he does through his work with the foundation. However, he must balance the needs of the foundation and its public health mission with the needs of his patient, "A physician shall, while caring for a patient, regard responsibility to the patient as paramount" (Principle VIII).

As a means of achieving the goals of both respecting his patient's rights and contributing to the betterment of public health, Dr. M could have engaged in a brainstorming session with the other board members and generated a list of celebrities whom they could invite to be involved with the foundation's fund-raiser. Famous older persons, like those who are not well known, seek mental health services. Despite natural temptations to the contrary, care must be taken by clinicians to not reveal the identities of famous patients or put them in positions that could be exploitative. Additionally, if famous patients become aware that their mental health provider is involved with a charitable organizations or activity, and then volunteer their name or presence as a way of helping the charity, the clinician should examine the patient's motivations and carefully consider the possible impact of such involvement on the therapeutic relationship and the patient's treatment before accepting the offer.

CASE 12

Father G provides religious services and counsels residents and their families in a long-term care facility. It has been his impression in recent years that, despite the seemingly unending barrage of new safety regulations, there have been increasing numbers of complaints from family members about injuries that their loved ones sustained from falls. Many of the falls seem to have occurred when residents became tired of waiting for assistance to transfer out of bed or from their wheelchair to the toilet and tried to do it themselves. Father G has observed that the increased number of falls corresponds with a decrease in the number of staff. Recently, instead of spending most of his time working with residents on late-life or end-of-life issues, he has been supporting family members who feel guilty both for being unable to care for their loved ones at home and for having placed them in a facility that has not kept them safe. In addition to the feelings of guilt and regret, the family members are angry at the facility's staff and administration.

DISCUSSION

When residents are admitted to long-term care facilities, it is with the explicit or implicit promise that the facility will keep the person safe (beneficence and nonmaleficence). Rules and regulations exist, staff members are trained, the physical environment is kept free of debris and safety hazards, and all manner of alarms, seat belts, and other safety devices are available to prevent falls, aggressive acts, unsafe transfers, and other causes of injury. Often, the residents or their family members have chosen a long-term care facility precisely because the residents have proven that they are unsafe at home. They want safety, and they are essentially assured, "Come to our facility, and we will keep you safe." However, no facility has a perfect safety record. No facility can fulfill the promise and the expectation. Despite the rational understanding by residents and/or family members that 100% safety is impossible, injuries to residents may engender in family members a belief that they were deceived. Family members in such situations often respond with anger and blaming.

When venting their frustrations and anger, family members often seek a sympathetic ear. Mental health professionals and clergy serve valuable functions through emotional support and education of disillusioned and angry residents and family members. However, clinicians and clergy in such contexts often have the seemingly daunting task of supporting family members without siding with them, except perhaps in extreme circumstances, against the facility. Pastoral counselors understand the importance of maintaining appropriate roles and relationships. While being sensitive to the frustrations of residents and their families, pastoral counselors do not malign other professionals (American Association of Pastoral Counselors, 1994, Principle II, I). Pastoral counselors and other mental health professionals who are able to demonstrate understanding and caring, while maintaining a position of neutrality on matters of fault, can serve as a valuable link between the resident/family and the staff or administrators who are perceived as being responsible for the injuries.

To facilitate the transition to long-term care facilities for older adults and their families, geriatric mental health professionals may elect to assist with public education and advocacy efforts. Many media outlets and opportunities are available to disseminate realistic information about long-term care to older adults, as well as to help correct widespread dissemination of misinformation. Advocacy can take many forms, including striving to change local policies or regulations to becoming involved in state or Federal legislative activities. These efforts may ultimately help to improve long-term care and better prepare consumers for the experience.

Learning Exercise

1. Describe an example of a situation involving a geriatric mental health professional that has societal implications. Use the decision-making model to determine ways to correct or improve the situation involving the clinician.

Conclusions

Mental health professionals utilize a wide variety of clinical skills across diverse practice contexts in the provision of care and service to older adults. Each service provided and each practice context involves both common and unique ethical issues and challenges. Despite the professional, ethical, and legal challenges, providing mental health services to older adults can be extremely rewarding, both personally and professionally. The satisfaction derived from working with older adults is maximized when clinicians anticipate and proactively address the ethical challenges that are likely to arise in their practice settings. However, many ethical dilemmas are not easily avoided or resolved, even by the most ethically conscious and well-intentioned clinicians.

There are times when ethical dilemmas tax the morality of both the professional and the profession. As Beauchamp and Childress (2001) stated, "No moral theorist or professional code of ethics has successfully presented a system of moral rules free of conflicts and exceptions, but this fact is not cause for either skepticism or alarm" (p. 15). Mental health professionals who possess the clinical and ethical competence to work with older adults are particularly well-equipped to address the myriad ethical conflicts and exceptions that may be encountered.

Geriatric mental health professionals have multiple professional, ethical, and legal obligations that exist to protect and promote the interests and well-being of older adult patients, families and other caregivers, and the public. Practitioners must strive to "advocate for an ethic for elderly that respects their dignity but also afford them the protection they deserve" (Hays, 1999, p. 662). When trying to balance the potentially competing demands of respecting dignity and providing protection, clinicians must consider the fit between their personal beliefs and values and the settings in which they work, and they must strive to anticipate and directly address ethical challenges.

Ethical decision-making models help provide a context in which ethical challenges can be understood and good solutions can be generated. Such models provide structure for organizing thoughts, resources, and options, so that clinicians can make good decisions based on relevant laws, ethical directives and principles, and their own values. Yet, despite the value of models, the mandates of codes, and the availability of numerous resources, "often what counts most in the moral life is not consistent adherence to principles and rules, but reliable character, good moral sense, and emotional responsiveness" (Beauchamp & Childress, 2001, p. 26). The development of a culture of professional and ethical responsibility within the workplace promotes sound clinical practice and satisfaction for patients, families, and clinicians.

The maintenance of ethical competence requires an ongoing commitment to increasing one's (a) understanding of ethical and legal issues encountered in geriatric mental health practice, (b) familiarity with an ethical decision-making model, (c) appreciation of the multiple resources that facilitate ethical decision making, and (d) personal investment in pursuing the highest ethical ideals. Geriatric mental health professionals will benefit from regularly including ethical and legal issues among their inservice and grand rounds topics.

Through the ethical provision of mental health services, we have the privilege and responsibility of providing improved understanding of the psychological, neurocognitive, social, and spiritual strengths and limitations associated with older adulthood. We have the honor and obligation to provide and promote older adults' treatment and care. And, by virtue of our knowledge, training, and experience, we are well positioned to provide advocacy on behalf of older adults and their loved ones. The need is growing; are we ready?

Americans are living longer. Despite multiple, serious chronic illnesses, millions survive into their ninth decade and beyond. Advances in medical technology and pharmacology have made clinical care of the elderly more demanding and decision making increasingly complex. At the same time, new ethical challenges confront practitioners caring for the aging population on a day-to-day basis.

Geriatric Mental Health Ethics: A Casebook is an important guide to assist readers facing these ethically demanding situations. The opening chapters describe common mental health problems in the elderly and define the fundamental principles of ethics-based practice. Subsequent chapters emphasize the connection between clinical and ethical decision making, as well as underscore the conflicts of legal and ethical matters. In the final chapters, an ethical decision-making model is proposed and demonstrated by case illustrations in eight aspects of practice applicable to a variety of disciplines and clinical settings.

The casebook is not a comprehensive review of all ethical principles governing every aspect of geriatric mental health care. The book's genuine value is that it provides the reader with a solid foundation in ethical competence. The 10-step ethical decision-making model described is a clear, structured roadmap to aid in the resolution of common ethical problems. The mental health practitioner may utilize this model in ethical decision making in much the same manner a clinician employs practice guidelines/algorithms or differential diagnosis methods. Arguably, this approach may be used not only in geriatric mental health practice, but in any clinical setting where ethical conflicts and concerns arise.

Most health care professionals receive little or no formal education or training in ethics-based practice. This casebook will be an invaluable resource to students in a multitude of clinical disciplines. Because of the volume's easy-to-read style and practical nature, seasoned practitioners will also find it to be of value in their busy clinical environments.

Geriatric Mental Health Ethics: A Casebook clearly achieves the goals set forth by its author. Ethical challenges in the elderly are described, available resources for ethical decision making are reviewed, and a template for discussion and resolution of ethical conundrums is demonstrated. Readers may apply the knowledge obtained in this casebook to provide competent ethical care in their everyday practice. *Geriatric Mental Health Ethics: A Casebook* is a welcome resource to all geriatric mental health students, practitioners, and educators.

Frank A. Cervo, MD, CMD
Medical Director
Long Island State Veterans Home
Associate Professor of Clinical Medicine
Stony Brook University School of Medicine

Selected Guidelines Relevant to Geriatric Mental Health

- Alexopoulos, G. S., Katz, I. R., Reynolds, C. F., Carpenter, D., & Docherty, J. P. (2001). *The Expert Consensus Guidelines^{TM}: Pharmacotherapy of depressive disorders in older patients.* A Postgraduate Medicine Special Report. The McGraw-Hill Companies, Inc. (www.psychguides.com/depression).
- Alexopoulos, G. S., Streim, J., Carpenter, D., & Docherty, J. P. (2004). The Expert Consensus Guidelines™: Using antipsychotic agents in older patients. *Journal of Clinical Psychiatry, 65(Suppl 2),* 1–105 (www.psychguides.com/ecgs14.php).
- American Association for Geriatric Psychiatry. (1997). *Psychotherapeutic Medication in the Nursing Home* (www.aagponline.org/prof/position_medication.asp).
- American Association for Geriatric Psychiatry. (2001). *Family and Caregiver Counseling in Dementia: Medical Necessity* (www.aagponline.org/prof/position_dementia.asp).
- American Association for Geriatric Psychiatry. (2001). *End-of-Life Care* (www.aagponline.org/prof/position_end.asp).

All references retrieved January 5, 2008.

- American Association for Geriatric Psychiatry. (2002). *Mental Health and Medical Care of Older Adults* (www.aagponline.org/prof/position_mental.asp).
- American Association for Geriatric Psychiatry. (2005). *Principles of Care for Patients with Dementia Resulting from Alzheimer Disease* (www.aagponline.org/prof/position_caredmnalz.asp).
- American Bar Association & American Psychological Association. (2005). *Assessment of Older Adults with Diminished Capacity: A Handbook for Lawyers* (www.apa.org/pi/aging/diminished_capacity.pdf).
- American Bar Association, American Psychological Association, & National College of Probate Judges. (2006). *Judicial Determination of Capacity of Older Adults in Guardianship Proceedings* (www.abanet.org/aging/docs/judges_book_5–24.pdf).
- American Geriatrics Society. (1993). *Mental Health and the Elderly* (www.americangeriatrics.org/products/positionpapers/mentalhl.shtml).
- American Geriatrics Society. (2002). *Making Treatment Decisions for Incapacitated Elderly Patients Without Advance Directives* (www.americangeriatrics.org/products/positionpapers/treatdec.shtml).
- American Geriatrics Society & American Association for Geriatric Psychiatry. (2003). *Recommendations for Policies in Support of Quality Mental Health Care in U.S. Nursing Homes* (www.americangeriatrics.org/education/policies2003.pdf).
- American Medical Directors Association. (2003). *Depression*. Columbia (MD): Author (www.guideline.gov/summary/summary.aspx?doc_id=4952&nbr=003520&string=geriatric+AND+mental+AND+health).
- American Medical Directors Association. (2005). *Pharmacotherapy companion to the depression clinical practice guideline*. Columbia, MD: Author (www.guideline.gov/summary/summary.aspx?doc_id=7509&nbr=004447&string=geriatric+AND+mental+AND+health).
- American Psychiatric Association. (1999). Practice guideline

for the treatment of patients with delirium. *American Journal of Psychiatry, 156(5 Suppl)*, 1–20 (www.guideline.gov/summary/summary.aspx?doc_id=2180&nbr=001406&string=geriatric+AND+mental+AND+health).

■ American Psychiatric Association. (2007). *Practice Guideline for the Treatment of Patients with Alzheimer's Disease and Other Dementias* (2nd ed.) (www.psych.org/psych_pract/treatg/pg/AlzPG101007.pdf).

■ American Psychological Association. (1998). *Guidelines for the Evaluation of Dementia and Age-Related Cognitive Decline* (apa.org/practice/dementia.html).

■ American Psychological Association. (2004). *Guidelines for Psychological Practice with Older Adults* (www.apa.org/practice/adult.pdf).

■ American Psychological Association Online. (2006). *Mental Health Care and Older Adults: Facts and Policy Recommendations* (www.apa.org/ppo/issues/oldermhfact03.html).

■ Arizona Department of Health Services, Division of Behavioral Health Services. (2007). *Older Adults: Behavioral Health Prevention, Early Intervention, and Treatment* (www.azdhs.gov/bhs/guidance/olderadult.pdf).

■ Bergman-Evans, B. (2004). *Improving medication management for older adult clients.* Iowa City, IA: University of Iowa Gerontological Nursing Interventions Research Center, Research Dissemination Core (www.guideline.gov/summary/summary.aspx?doc_id=6222&nbr=003993&string=geriatric+AND+mental+AND+health).

■ Brown, E. L., Raue, P. J., & Halpert, K. D. (2007). *Detection of depression in older adults with dementia.* Iowa City, IA: University of Iowa Gerontological Nursing Interventions Research Center, Research Dissemination Core (www.guideline.gov/summary/summary.aspx?doc_id=11054&nbr=005833&string=geriatric+AND+mental+AND+health).

■ California Workgroup on Guidelines for Alzheimer's Disease Management. (2002). *Guidelines for Alzheimer's disease management.* Los Angeles, CA: Alzheimer's Association of Los Angeles, Riverside and San Bernardino Counties (http://www.

guideline.gov/summary/summary.aspx?doc_id=3157&nbr= 002383&string=geriatric+AND+mental+AND+health).

- Daly, J. M. (2004). *Elder abuse prevention*. Iowa City, IA: University of Iowa Gerontological Nursing Interventions Research Center, Research Dissemination Core (www.guideline.gov/ summary/summary.aspx?doc_id=6829&nbr=004196&string= geriatric+AND+mental+AND+health).
- Foreman, M. D., Fletcher, K., Mion, L. C., & Trygstad, L. (2003). Assessing cognitive function. In M. Mezey, T. Fulmer, I. Abraham, & D. A. Zwicker (Eds.). *Geriatric nursing protocols for best practice* (2nd ed., pp. 99–115). New York: Springer Publishing Company, Inc. (www.guideline.gov/summary/summary. aspx?doc_id=3508&nbr=002734&string=geriatric+AND+ mental+AND+health).
- Foreman, M. D., Mion, L. C., Trygstad, L., & Fletcher, K. (2003). Delirium: Strategies for assessing and treating. In M. Mezey, T. Fulmer, I. Abraham, & D. A. Zwicker (Eds.), *Geriatric nursing protocols for best practice* (2nd ed., pp. 116–140). New York: Springer Publishing Company, Inc. (www.guideline. gov/summary/summary.aspx?doc_id=3509&nbr=002735 &string=geriatric+AND+mental+AND+health).
- Gaskamp, C. D., Sutter, R., & Meraviglia, M. (2004). *Promoting spirituality in the older adult*. Iowa City, IA: University of Iowa Gerontological Nursing Interventions Research Center, Research Dissemination Core (www.guideline.gov/summary/ summary.aspx?doc_id=6830&nbr=004197&string=geriatric+ AND+mental+AND+health).
- Herr, K., Bjoro, K., Steffensmeier, J., & Rakel, B. (2006). *Acute pain management in older adults*. Iowa City, IA: University of Iowa Gerontological Nursing Interventions Research Center, Research Translation and Dissemination Core (www.guideline. gov/summary/summary.aspx?doc_id=10198&nbr=005382 &string=geriatric+AND+mental+AND+health).
- Institute for Clinical Systems Improvement. (2007). *Major depression in adults in primary care*. Bloomington, MN: Institute for Clinical Systems Improvement (www.guideline.gov/

summary/summary.aspx?doc_id=10866&nbr=005679&string
=geriatric+AND+mental+AND+health).

- Knopman, D. S., DeKosky, S. T., Cummings, J. L., Chui, H.,
  Corey-Bloom, J., Relkin, N., Small, G. W., Miller, B., & Stevens,
  J. C. (2001). Practice parameter: Diagnosis of dementia (an
  evidence-based review): Report of the quality standards sub-
  committee of the American Academy of Neurology. *Neurology*,
  56, 1143–1153 (www.guideline.gov/summary/summary.aspx?
  doc_id=2817&nbr=002043&string=geriatric+AND+mental
  +AND+health).

- Kurlowicz, L. H. (2003). Depression in older adults. In M.
  Mezey, T. Fulmer, I. Abraham, & D. A. Zwicker (Eds.), *Geriatric nursing protocols for best practice*. (2nd ed., pp. 185–206).
  New York: Springer Publishing Company, Inc. (www.guideline.
  gov/summary/summary.aspx?doc_id=3512&nbr=002738
  &string=geriatric+AND+mental+AND+health).

- Meraviglia, M., Sutter, R., & Gaskamp, C. D. (2006). *Providing
  spiritual care to the terminally ill older adult*. Iowa City, IA: University of Iowa Gerontological Nursing Interventions Research
  Center, Research Dissemination Core (www.guideline.gov/
  summary/summary.aspx?doc_id=10552&nbr=005515&string
  =geriatric+AND+mental+AND+health).

- Michigan Quality Improvement Consortium. (2005). *Screening
  and management of substance use disorders*. Southfield, MI:
  Michigan Quality Improvement Consortium (www.guideline.
  gov/summary/summary.aspx?doc_id=8161&nbr=004548
  &string=geriatric+AND+mental+AND+health).

- National Association of Social Workers. (2007). *Long-term care*
  (www.americangeriatrics.org/products/positionpapers/treatdec.
  shtml).

- Petersen, R. C., Stevens, J. C., Ganguli, M., Tangalos, E. G.,
  Cummings, J. L., & DeKosky, S. T. (2001). Practice parameter:
  Early detection of dementia: Mild cognitive impairment (an
  evidence-based review): Report of the Quality Standards Sub-
  committee of the American Academy of Neurology. *Neurology*,
  56, 1133–1142 (www.guideline.gov/summary/summary.aspx?

doc_id=2816&nbr=002042&string=geriatric+AND+mental +AND+health).

- Piven, M. L. S. (2005). *Detection of depression in the cognitively intact older adult.* Iowa City, IA: University of Iowa Gerontological Nursing Interventions Research Center, Research Dissemination Core (www.guideline.gov/summary/summary.aspx? doc_id=8112&nbr=004519&string=geriatric+AND+mental +AND+health).
- Registered Nurses Association of Ontario. (2003). *Screening for delirium, dementia and depression in older adults.* Toronto, ON: Registered Nurses Association of Ontario (www.guideline.gov/ summary/summary.aspx?doc_id=5313&nbr=003636&string= geriatric+AND+mental+AND+health).
- Registered Nurses Association of Ontario. (2004). *Caregiving strategies for older adults with delirium, dementia and depression.* Toronto, ON: Registered Nurses Association of Ontario (www.guideline.gov/summary/summary.aspx?doc_id=5737 &nbr=003848&string=geriatric+AND+mental+AND+ health).
- Umlauf, M. G., Chasens, E. R., & Weaver, T. E. (2003). Excessive sleepiness. In M. Mezey, T. Fulmer, I. Abraham, & D. A. Zwicker (Eds.), *Geriatric nursing protocols for best practice* (2nd ed., pp. 47–65). New York: Springer Publishing Company, Inc.   (www.guideline.gov/summary/summary.aspx?doc_id= 3505&nbr=002731&string=geriatric+AND+mental+AND+ health).
- University of Texas, School of Nursing. (2006). *Unintentional weight loss in the elderly.* Austin, TX: University of Texas, School of Nursing (www.guideline.gov/summary/summary.aspx.?doc_ id=9435&nbr=005056&string=geriatric+AND+mental+ AND+health).

Questionnaire of Surrogate Values

Name:_____Relation to patient:_____Date:_____

The following questions pertain to your values and beliefs about life and death in general.

1. T/F Living a long life is extremely important to me.
2. T/F Living a productive, rewarding, and meaningful life is extremely important to me.
3. T/F Being physically comfortable is extremely important to me.
4. T/F Being treated with dignity and respect is extremely important to me.
5. T/F Being independent is extremely important to me.
6. T/F I trust my family.
   Specify exceptions:
7. T/F Being with family is important to me.
   Specify exceptions:

This questionnaire is offered as a general template for helping to understand the values of surrogate decision makers, which may impact the decisions that are made for others, and is designed to facilitate discussion. It is not intended to be all-inclusive. It may benefit from further revision or study. The idea for the questionnaire was derived from the work of Doukas and McCullough (1988).

8. T/F   I am afraid of death.

9. T/F   I am afraid of dying.

10. T/F   I am not afraid of dying if my pain is limited.

The following questions pertain to your values and beliefs about living for more than 6 months without the ability to make decisions for yourself.

11. T/F   Living as long as possible is extremely important to me, even if it means having a poor quality of life.

12. T/F   I would rather die than live with considerable pain or other discomfort.

13. T/F   I would rather die than live with significantly decreased dignity and respect.

14. T/F   I would rather die than be kept alive artificially (e.g., feeding tube, respirator, endotracheal tube), even if I do not appear to be in pain.

15. T/F   I would rather die than be dependent on others for basic needs, such as eating and toileting.

16. T/F   I would rather die than live without the ability to make medical decisions for myself.

17. T/F   I would trust my family members to make decisions that are in my best interests if I am unable to do so.

18. T/F   I would welcome family involvement in my life if I were so impaired that I required total assistance for basic needs such as feeding and toileting.

19. T/F   If a determination is made, based on my values, not to artificially prolong my life, family members and friends should take comfort in the fact that I am not afraid of death or dying.

20. T/F   I would rather die with/without pain relief from medications than live in a significantly compromised medical state.

Other comments:
_____

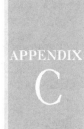

Answers to Learning Exercises

CHAPTER 1

1. b. He, Sengupta, Velkoff, and DeBarros (2005) found that depressive symptoms affect approximately 15% of community-dwelling older adults and up to 25% of those in nursing homes.
2. d. Older adulthood inevitably includes loss.
3. False. Fortunately, like previous developmental stages, older adulthood does offer opportunities for personal growth and changes that enrich life.

CHAPTER 2

1. The specific responses to this learning exercise may vary between clinicians because of differences in practice contexts, differences in resources provided by the various professions, and the specificity of jurisdictional laws that govern the practice of the various professions. As a psychologist providing services

to older adults, the top 5 resources that I would typically consider in order to avoid or resolve an ethical dilemma are as follows:

1. Jurisdictional laws
2. *Ethical Principles of Psychologists and Code of Conduct* (American Psychological Association, 2002)
3. Professional guidelines and scholarly publications pertaining to ethical practice
4. Experienced and ethically knowledgeable colleagues
5. Principle-based bioethical principles

The resources that I include on my list and the order in which I rank them are flexible. For example, if I anticipated that the ethical problem could result in a complaint against me with the state licensing board or an ethics committee, my list of resources would be topped by my professional liability insurance carrier and an attorney. In other instances, a quick conversation or E-mail exchange with a respected colleague may suffice.

2. Values that are shared by members of a society, such as the right of competent adults to make the decisions that govern their lives, are reflected in general bioethical principles. These values and principles are then typically adopted, explicitly or implicitly, by the medical and mental health professions of the society and underlie the ethical principles that guide professional behavior.

Thus, professional codes of ethics are based on the shared values of a profession for the protection and promotion of the welfare of patients, the profession, and society. Professional ethics reflect the common morality or values of the larger society.

CHAPTER 3

1. d. The Older Americans Act (a) reinforces the American value of dignity as an inherent right of older adults, (b) establishes entitlements to which older adults must have an equal

opportunity for full and free enjoyment, and (c) tasks the U.S. government with duties and responsibilities to promote the dignity of older Americans. However, the Older Americans Act does not mandate that by the year 2015 all U.S. sidewalks have curb cuts so that they are wheelchair accessible.

2. c. Skilled nursing facilities became a ready alternative to psychiatric hospitals for older adults with serious mental illness during the movement in the U.S. to deinstitutionalize psychiatric inpatients.

3. False. When surveyed by Pope, Tabachnick, and Keith-Spiegel (1987) and Gibson and Pope (1993), mental health professionals reported that when they are engaged in ethical decision making, they prefer to turn first to their professional ethics code and the perspectives of colleagues whereas laws, scholarly ethics publications, and local ethics committees were among those resources valued least.

CHAPTER 4

1. True. Pope and Vetter (1992) found that psychologists, in general, are most concerned about confidentiality issues, with concerns about professional competence ranked 11th. In contrast, Bush (2007) reported that neuropsychologists are most concerned about professional competence, with confidentiality concerns ranked 5th.

2. The specific responses to this learning exercise will vary because of differences in clinical activities between professions, differences in the nature and context of practices within and between professions, and individual differences in ethical issues that are considered most concerning given the unique aspects of our professional activities. In my independent practice, I find the following ethical issues to be most challenging:

    1. Third-party requests for services: Having services initiated by a patient's family members can raise complex issues regarding who is involved in the evaluation and/or treatment and who will receive feedback about the patient's status.

2. Privacy and confidentiality: As noted previously, having close family members or caregivers present while services are provided or having them interested in information obtained or conveyed during sessions can become problematic if the nature and limits of confidentiality are not clarified at the outset of the services and as needed thereafter.

3. Informed consent: Many of the potential problems associated with third-party requests for services and privacy/confidentiality can be avoided or readily resolved if these issues are handled appropriately during the informed consent process. However, expectations that all foreseeable problems can be addressed at the outset are not reasonable. I must attempt to identify and address during the informed consent process those points that may be reasonably identified as potentially problematic if neglected.

4. Use of assessments: Many older adults have sensory, motor, or other limitations that require modifications to standardized test administration. The applicability of normative data in such situations can be problematic, which raises questions about whether and in which circumstances such modifications should be applied and how the results should be interpreted.

5. Bases for scientific and professional judgments: As noted previously, the results of standardized assessment measures upon which psychologists often rely may not be a valid representation of the construct being assessed. As a result, more subjective clinical impressions and judgments may necessarily replace more evidence-based conclusions. A conservative approach to clinical determinations is needed in such instances. Additionally, family members and others involved in patients' lives may, for a variety of reasons, attempt to influence my opinions. I must make a concerted effort in such situations to not let external pressures influence my clinical decision making.

3. The specific responses to this learning exercise will vary for the same reasons described above. In my practice and location, I am most concerned about the following threats to ethical

practice by my colleagues, most of which can be harmful to patients or others or, at best, are not beneficial:

1. Competence: Some of the written work generated by colleagues (e.g., test reports) that I have the opportunity to review suggests less than adequate competence to provide services to older adults. Such work has a high likelihood of being harmful, in some manner, to patients.

2. Integrity and justice: Some colleagues that I know to be competent, nevertheless, arrive at conclusions that are not based on available science. Often, I encounter compromised integrity in forensic contexts in which clinicians arrive at conclusions that favor the retaining party regardless of the accuracy or truthfulness of the clinician's conclusions. Integrity is also of concern in situations in which clinicians know that they lack the necessary education and training to provide competent services, but they do so anyway, often motivated by personal financial gain.

3. Multiple relationships: Clinicians who perform forensic evaluations of patients with whom they have treating relationships have created or accepted a multiple relationship, and there is a strong likelihood that both their forensic determinations and the therapeutic relationship will be adversely affected.

4. Record keeping: There are some clinicians in my region whose record keeping is insufficient to allow review by colleagues and payors and is inconsistent with established ethical requirements (Ethical Standard 6.01 Documentation of Professional and Scientific Work and Maintenance of Records; American Psychological Association, 2002) and professional guidelines (American Psychological Association, 2007).

5. Bases for scientific and professional judgments: Whether the result of insufficient competence or compromised integrity, some clinicians offer impressions and conclusions regarding diagnosis, prognosis, and disability status that are not based on available scientific evidence.

CHAPTER 5

1. Prior to entering Mr. A's room, Brian should have informed the nursing staff that he would be conducting an intake interview and that it would be important to avoid interruptions. Placing a "do not disturb" sign on the door would also help promote privacy. Once in the patient's/resident's room, it is typically preferable to directly address the patient/resident unless there is a good reason not to do so, such as advanced knowledge that the resident has significant comprehension or cognitive problems. After initial introductions and a description of his role, Brian should have taken Mr. A to a private setting, such as Brian's office, or asked Mr. A's family members and the roommate's wife to leave the room until the intake interview had been completed. Depending on the roommate's mobility, he should also be asked to leave the room, or efforts should be made to maximize Mr. A's privacy with the roommate present, such as drawing the curtain between the beds and speaking in a lowered voice (as long as Mr. A could adequately hear what was being said). Such efforts would have promoted privacy and confidentiality.

CHAPTER 6

1. The specific responses to this learning exercise will likely vary between members of different mental health professions because of the differences in their education, training, and scopes of practice. However, the answer should include, at a minimum, (a) broad-based education in the core requirements of the discipline, (b) coursework specific to biopsychosocial issues in later adulthood, and (c) supervised training in the provision of clinical services to older adults.

   For someone interested in becoming a psychologist who provides clinical services to older adults, I would recommend (a) pursuit of doctorate in clinical or counseling psychology, with the broad-based education associated with such programs;

(b) elective coursework in areas related to geriatric practice (see, for example, the *Guidelines for Psychological Practice with Older Adults*; American Psychological Association, 2004); (c) completion of a dissertation or PsyD project related to geropsychology; (d) supervised predoctoral practicum and internship experience with older adults; and (e) postdoctoral fellowship in geropsychology. Completion of such education and training should establish an entry level of professional competence needed to provide clinical services to older adults. Attainment of the generalist licensure to practice independently should be followed by continuing education courses and informal consultation.

I also recommend that, once eligible, clinicians undergo a formal peer review process in the form of board certification. Although the American Board of Professional Psychology does not currently offer board certification in the specialty of geriatric psychology, psychologists who provide clinical services to older adults can pursue board certification in clinical psychology and emphasize their work with older adults in their work samples and oral examination. Additionally, psychologists who work primarily with older adults in specific contexts (e.g., physical medicine and rehabilitation) or provide more specialized services (e.g., neuropsychological services) may pursue board certification through one of these specialties.

2. First, I would begin to educate myself about practice in the new setting. I would carefully consider the nature of the patients and the services to be provided. I would review the job description, if one is available, or draft a description of my new responsibilities as I understood them. I would then begin reading relevant books, journal articles, and other resources that would help prepare me to provide competent services in the new setting.

   Second, I would pursue additional formal education at whatever level was necessary to ensure my competence to practice in the new setting. Such education may consist of continuing education courses or completion of a formal respecialization program.

Third, I would obtain peer consultation or supervision. I may pursue this step first to clarify the expectations inherent in the new setting. The opportunity to discuss cases with a colleague experienced in the setting that I am entering would be essential prior to and/or during the transition. The reasons for the transition and amount of time available prior to the change will influence the timing and nature of the preparations that may be made for such a transition.

CHAPTER 7

1. I would strongly recommend to the woman that she consider psychotherapy to explore her thoughts and feelings about her situation, including her medical status, her surgical options, and her initial choice to forego life saving surgery. I would want her to fully consider the impact of her decision on her love ones. If I were to provide the psychotherapy, I would examine my own beliefs and values regarding the woman's situation and decision and strive to not impose my values on her.

    With regard to the surgeon, I would inform him that the woman was indeed competent to make medical decisions for herself. I would acknowledge, although not necessarily explicitly state to the surgeon, his wish to keep the woman alive and his frustration with her decision to let the disease take her life. I would inform him of the woman's decision about undergoing psychotherapy and, if she had accepted the offer of psychotherapy, reassure the surgeon that she may very well change her mind once she has had more time to reflect on her options and their implications.

CHAPTER 8

1. *Privacy* refers to the right of individuals to choose how much of their personal information may be shared with others. Privacy is a fundamental human right; it is essential to ensure one's

dignity and freedom of self-determination (Koocher & Keith-Spiegel, 1998) and is based on the principle of respect for autonomy (Beauchamp & Childress, 2001).

Confidentiality is based on the right to privacy and poses limits on the release of patient information to others.

Privilege is defined as "a right or immunity granted as a peculiar benefit, advantage, or favor" (Merriam-Webster, 1988, p. 936). Privilege relieves the clinician from having to testify in court about a patient's communications; thus, it is a narrower concept than confidentiality.

2. The right to be fully informed regarding proposed mental health services and to consent to, or decline, participation as a result of that information is based on the bioethical principle of respect for autonomy.

3. Obtaining descriptions of the patient's values from two or more sources can increase the reliability of the information. Additionally, obtaining a description of the surrogate's values and comparing that information to the patient's values can help clarify whether the surrogate's decisions are more reflective of his or her values or the values of the patient. The *Questionnaire of Surrogate Values* provided in Appendix B can facilitate this process.

CHAPTER 9

1. For a variety of reasons, such as sensory and motor deficits, clinicians at times cannot administer tests in the manner in which they were standardized. When the characteristics of a given patient require the clinician to diverge from standardized administration, thus limiting the extent to which normative data can be used in the interpretation of the test results, clinicians must carefully consider whether performing the testing with accommodations will result in informative or misleading findings. There are many instances in which valuable information about a construct of interest (e.g., memory) can be obtained

despite having to modify the test administration because of sensory or motor deficits. Clinicians who administer standardized tests to older adults must develop skill in tailoring evaluations to accommodate both the specific characteristics of the patient and the context in which the evaluation is performed, and they must temper their conclusions accordingly.

Additionally, clinicians must seek published studies that provide information about the modifications that they are considering. For example, when assessing the visuoconstructional abilities of persons with hemiparesis of their dominant (typically right) side, it would be valuable to review the studies performed by Bush (2000a and 2000b) and colleagues (Bush & Martin, 2004b) to determine whether having the patients complete the tests with their nondominant hand would result in valid information about the construct of interest (i.e., visuoconstructional ability).

CHAPTER 10

1. a. As stated in the Preamble to the American Medical Association's Principles of Medical Ethics, the doctor's/clinician's *primary* responsibility is to his or her patients.
2. d. Older adult men have the highest rate of suicide.
3. d. No single psychotherapeutic treatment modality has emerged as superior to others in the treatment of older adults. The possession of specialized skills in treating older adults supersedes any single treatment modality.

CHAPTER 11

1. The specific responses to this learning exercise will likely vary considerably because of differences in practice contexts and patient populations. The important point is that sensitivity to, and understanding of, cultural and disability issues must be

promoted in our practices and the practices of our colleagues. Particular attention should be paid to the potential impact of these issues on the mental health services provided to a given individual.

Hinrichsen (2006) advised three primary steps to help mental health professionals establish competence with combined multicultural and aging issues: Learn more, teach more, and talk more. Mental health professionals who work with disabled, diverse, or otherwise unique older adult populations have a responsibility to initiate conversations with colleagues, trainees, caregivers, and others about these complex issues. Such conversation is a primary and ongoing step toward maximizing the care, treatment, and well-being of older adult patients.

CHAPTER 12

1. For a variety of reasons, there is no single answer that applies universally to this question; nevertheless, the question is important for clinicians to consider in the context of their own practices. First, "interventions" come in many forms, and the nature and degree of empirical support needed to be considered "sufficient" for one intervention may be more or less than that needed for another intervention. For example, a pharmacological intervention may require more studies and more rigorous study designs compared to some psychotherapeutic interventions because the risks associated with medications are often greater than the risks associated with psychotherapy. Second, because of the differences among the various psychotherapeutic approaches, they do not lend themselves equally to scientific scrutiny. For example, some approaches may lend themselves more readily to quantifiable variables and statistical analyses, whereas others tend to be examined more through pseudoscientific methods such as case studies. Third, some patient populations or diagnoses, or combinations of patients and diagnoses, may prove difficult to study, resulting in very few studies involving persons that are similar to a given

patient. Thus, clinicians must determine whether they believe that there is sufficient evidence to support employing a given intervention with a specific patient, with the understanding that in some contexts their decisions will be critically examined by third parties.

When mental health professionals consider recommending or providing treatments that are less well-established, it is particularly important to weigh the potential benefits against the potential risks and costs and to involve the patient or the surrogate decision maker in the decision-making process. The use of innovative treatments is consistent with ethical practice in those instances in which the potential costs and risks are minimal (nonmaleficence), the potential for benefit exists (beneficence), expectations can be carefully managed, and patients or their surrogates provide informed consent (respect for autonomy).

2. The answer to this question depends on the therapist's values and, to some extent, the therapeutic approach. My approach is to facilitate an examination of the patient's perspective on aging, in general and with regard to the patient's life, while minimizing, to the extent possible, the introduction of my personal values into the therapeutic process. Some clinicians may argue that an approach of therapeutic neutrality and value neutrality with regard to aging is neither possible nor advisable, but the approach reflects my education, training, and personal preference and seems appropriate for most of the patients seen in my practice.

CHAPTER 13

1. Readers should generate their own examples for this learning exercise and then outline and resolve the issues using the ethical decision-making model. The cases presented in chapter 13 provide good examples of the types of issues that have societal influences or implications.

References

Ables, N. (2006, Spring). Competency in and with older adults. *The Register Report*, 32–35.

American Academy of Clinical Neuropsychology (AACN). (2007). Practice guidelines for neuropsychological assessment and consultation. *The Clinical Neuropsychologist, 21*, 209–231.

American Association of Pastoral Counselors. (1994). *Code of ethics*. Retrieved May 13, 2008, from www.aapc.org/ethics.cfm

American Bar Association Commission on Law and Aging & American Psychological Association. (2005). *Assessment of older adults with diminished capacity: A handbook for lawyers*. Washington, DC: Author.

American Counseling Association. (2005). *Code of ethics*. Retrieved April 22, 2008, from www.counseling.org/Resources/CodeOfEthics/TP/Home/CT2.aspx

American Educational Research Association, American Psychological Association, National Council on Measurement in Education. (1999). *Standards for educational and psychological testing*. Washington, DC: American Educational Research Association.

American Geriatrics Society. (2008). *Frequently asked questions about geriatricians and the shortage of geriatrics healthcare providers*. Retrieved March 16, 2008, from www.americangeriatrics.org/news/geria_faqs.shtml

American Medical Association, Council on Ethical and Judicial Affairs. (2006). *Code of Medical ethics of the American Medical Association, current opinions with annotations* (2006–2007 ed.). Washington, DC: Author.

American Mental Health Counselors Association. (2000). *Code of Ethics*. Retrieved September 1, 2007, from www.amhca.org/code

American Psychiatric Association. (2001). *Opinions of the ethics committee on the principles of medical ethics with annotations especially applicable to psychiatry*. Washington, DC: Author.

American Psychiatric Association. (2006). *The principles of medical ethics with annotations especially applicable to psychiatry*. Retrieved April 22, 2008, from www.psych.org/MainMenu/PsychiatricPractice/Ethics/ResourcesStandards/PrinciplesofMedical Ethics.aspx

American Psychological Association. (2002a). Ethical principles of psychologists and code of conduct. *American Psychologist, 57*, 1060–1073.

American Psychological Association. (2002b). *Guidelines on multicultural education, training, research, practice, and organizational change for psychologists*. Retrieved April 22, 2008, from www.apa.org/pi/multiculturalguidelines/homepage.html

American Psychological Association. (2003). *Depression and suicide in older adults resource guide*. Retrieved May 28, 2004, from http://www.apa.org/pi/aging/depression. html

American Psychological Association. (2004). Guidelines for psychological practice with older adults. *American Psychologist, 59* (4), 236–260.

American Psychological Association. (2007). Record keeping guidelines. *American Psychologist, 62*, 993–1004.

American Psychological Association, Presidential Task Force on the Assessment of Age-Consistent Memory Decline and Dementia. (1998). *Guidelines for the evaluation of dementia and age-related cognitive decline*. Washington, DC: American Psychological Association.

American Psychological Association, Working Group on Assisted Suicide and End-of-Life Decisions. (2000). *Report of the board of directors of APA from the Working Group on Assisted Suicide and End-of-Life Decisions*. Retrieved May 28, 2004, from http://www.apa.org/pi/aseol/section1.html

American Psychological Association Working Group on the Older Adult. (1998). What practitioners should know about working with older adults. *Professional Psychology: Research and Practice, 29*, 413–427.

Americans with Disabilities Act of 1990, Public Law Number 101–336, 104 Stat. 328 (1990).

Appelbaum, P. S. (2002). Privacy in psychiatric treatment: Threats and responses. *American Journal of Psychiatry, 159*, 1809–1818.

Ardern, M. (2004). Ethical aspects of psychotherapy and clinical work with older adults. In S. Evans & J. Garner (Eds.), *Talking over the years: A handbook of dynamic psychotherapy with older adults* (pp. 117–128). New York: Riutledge.

Association of Directors of Geriatric Academic Programs. (2007). *Status of geriatrics workforce study*. Retrieved March 16, 2008, from www.adgapstudy.uc.edu/Publications.cfm

Association of State and Provincial Psychology Boards. (2005). *Code of conduct*. Retrieved June 10, 2005, from www.asppb.org/publications/model/conduct.aspx

Baird, K. A., & Ruppert, P. A. (1987). Clinical management of confidentiality: A survey of psychologists in seven states. *Professional Psychology: Research and Practice, 18*, 347–352.

Balanced Budget Act of 1997. Pub.L. 105–33, 111 Stat. 251 (1997).

Ball, K., Berch, D. B., Helmers, K. F., Jobe, J. B., Leveck, M. D., Marsiske, M., et al. (2002). Effects of cognitive training interventions with older adults. *Journal of the American Medical Association, 288* (18), 2271–2281.

Barber v. Superior Court, 195 Cal Rptr 484, 147 Cal App 3d 1006 (1983).

Bartels, S. J. (Ed.) (2005). Evidence-based geriatric psychiatry. *Psychiatric Clinics of North America, 28*, 763–1122.

Bartels, S. J., Dums, A. R., Oxman, T. E., Schneider, L. S., Areán, P. A., Alexopoulos, G. S., et al. (2003). Evidence-based practices in geriatric mental health care: An overview of systematic reviews and meta-analyses. *Psychiatric Clinics of North America, 26*, 971–990, x–xi.

Beauchamp, T. L., & Childress, J. F. (2001). *Principles of biomedical ethics* (5th ed.). New York: Oxford University Press.

Beckingham, A. C., & Watts, S. (1995). Daring to grow old: Lessons in healthy aging and empowerment: Learning to live at all ages (Special issue). *Educational Gerontology, 21,* 479–495.

Behnke, S. H., Perlin, M. L., & Bernstein, M. (2003). *The essentials of New York Mental Health Law.* New York: W. W. Norton & Company.

Bennett, B. E., Bricklin, P. M., Harris, E., Knapp, S., VandeCreek, L., & Younggren, J. N. (2006). *Assessing and managing risk in psychological practice: An individualized approach.* Rockville, MD: The Trust.

Bentley, J. P., & Thacker, P. G. (2004). The influence of risk and monetary payment on the research participation decision making process. *Journal of Medical Ethics, 30,* 293–298.

Bersoff, D. N. (1999). Confidentiality, privilege, and privacy. In D. N. Bersoff (Ed.), *Ethical conflicts in psychology* (2nd ed., pp. 149–150). Washington, DC: American Psychological Association.

Bersoff, D., & Koeppl, P. (1993). The relations between ethical codes and moral principles. *Ethics and Behavior, 3,* 345–357.

Binder, L., & Thompson, L. (1995). The ethics code and neuropsychological assessment practices. *Archives of Clinical Neuropsychology, 10,* 27–46.

Binstock, R. H. (2004). Anti-aging medicine and research: A realm of conflict and profound societal implications. *The Journals of Gerontology Series A: Biological Sciences and Medical Sciences, 59,* B523–B533.

Blank, K. (2004) Legal and ethical issues. In J. Savdavoy, L. F. Jarrik, G. T. Grossberg, & S. M. Barnett (Eds.), *Comprehensive textbook of geriatric psychiatry* (3rd ed., pp. 1183–1206). New York: Norton & Co.

Blase, J. J. (2008). Trained third-party presence during forensic neuropsychological evaluations. In A. M. Horton, Jr., & D. Wedding (Eds.), *The neuropsychology handbook* (3rd ed., pp. 499–513). New York: Springer Publishing.

Bowers v. Hardwick, 478 U.S. 186. (1985).

Bowling, C. L. (1993). The concepts of successful and positive aging. *Family Practice, 10,* 449–453.

Bricklin, P. (2001). Being ethical: More than obeying the law and avoiding harm. *Journal of Personality Assessment, 77,* 195–202.

Brickman, A. M., Cabo, R., & Manly, J. J. (2006). Ethical issues in cross-cultural neuropsychology. *Applied Neuropsychology, 13,* 91–100.

Brittain, J. L., Frances, J. P., & Barth, J. T. (1995). Ethical issues and dilemmas in neuropsychological practice reported by ABCN diplomates. *Advances in Medical Psychotherapy, 8,* 1–22.

Brophy v. New England Sinai Hospital Inc., 497 NE 2d 626 (1986).

Browndyke, J. N. (2005). Ethical challenges with the use of information technology and telecommunications in neuropsychology, Part I. In S. S. Bush (Ed.), *A casebook of ethical challenges in neuropsychology.* (pp.179–198) New York: Psychology Press.

Bush, S. S. (2000a). Intermanual differences in performing a visuoconstructional task. *Archives of Physical Medicine and Rehabilitation, 81,* 1151–1152.

Bush, S. S. (2000b). Intermanual visuoconstruction differences in rehabilitation patients. *The Journal of Cognitive Rehabilitation, 18* (6), 10–12.

Bush, S. S. (2006). Neurocognitive enhancement: Ethical issues for an emerging subspecialty. *Applied Neuropsychology, 13* (2), 125–136.

Bush, S. S. (2007). *Ethical decision making in clinical neuropsychology*. New York: Oxford University Press.

Bush, S. S. (2008). Ethical cross-training in head trauma rehabilitation. *Journal of Head Trauma Rehabilitation, 23*, 181–184.

Bush, S. S. (in press). Legal and ethical considerations in rehabilitation and health assessment. In E. Mpofu & T. Oakland (Eds.), *Assessment in rehabilitation and health*. Boston: Allyn & Bacon.

Bush, S. S., Barth, J. T., Pliskin, N. H., Arffa, S., Axelrod, B. N., Blackburn, L. A., et al. (National Academy of Neuropsychology Policy & Planning Committee). (2005). Independent and court-ordered forensic neuropsychological examinations: Official statement of the National Academy of Neuropsychology. *Archives of Clinical Neuropsychology, 20* (8), 997–1007.

Bush, S. S., Connell, M. A., & Denney, R. L. (2006). *Ethical issues in forensic psychology: Key concepts and resources*. Washington, DC: American Psychological Association.

Bush, S. S., Grote, C., Johnson-Greene, D., & Macartney-Filgate, M. (2008). A panel interview on the ethical practice of neuropsychology. *The Clinical Neuropsychologist, 22*, 321-344.

Bush, S. S., & Martin, T. A. (2004a). *Balancing bioethical principles in computer-based memory treatment*. Poster presentation at the 9th International Conference on Alzheimer's Disease and Related Disorders. July 18, 2004, Philadelphia, PA.

Bush, S. S., & Martin, T. A. (2004b). Intermanual differences on the Rey Complex Figure Test. *Rehabilitation Psychology, 49* (1), 76–8.

Bush, S. S., & Martin, T. A. (2005). Ethical issues in geriatric neuropsychology. In S. S. Bush & T. A. Martin (Eds.), *Geriatric neuropsychology: Practice essentials* (pp. 507–536). New York: Psychology Press.

Bush, S. S., & Martin, T. A. (2008). Confidentiality in neuropsychological practice. In A. M. Horton, Jr. & D. Wedding (Eds.), *The Neuropsychology handbook* (3rd ed.). New York: Springer Publishing.

Bush, S. S., Grote, C., Johnson-Greene, D., & Macartney-Filgate, M. (2008). A panel interview on the ethical practice of neuropsychology. *The Clinical Neuropsychologist, 22*, 321–344.

Bush, S., Naugle, R., & Johnson-Greene, D. (2002). The interface of information technology and neuropsychology: Ethical issues and recommendations. *The Clinical Neuropsychologist, 16* (4), 536–547.

Bush, S. S., Ruff, R. M., Tröster, A. I., Barth, J. T., Koffler, S. P., Pliskin, N. H., et al. (National Academy of Neuropsychology Policy & Planning Committee), (2005). Symptom validity assessment: Practice issues and medical necessity. Official position of the National Academy of Neuropsychology. *Archives of Clinical Neuropsychology, 20*(4), 419–426.

Byrd, D. A., & Manly, J. J. (2005). Cultural considerations in neuropsychological assessment of older adults. In S. S. Bush & T. A. Martin (Eds.), *Geriatric neuropsychology: Practice essentials* (pp. 115–139). New York: Psychology Press.

Caplan, B., & Shechter, J. (2005). Test accommodations in geriatric neuropsychology. In S. S. Bush & T. A. Martin (Eds.), *Geriatric neuropsychology: Practice essentials* (pp. 97–114). New York: Psychology Press.

Cervo, F. A., Bryan, L., & Farber, S. (2006). To PEG or not PEG: A review of evidence for placing feeding tubes in advanced dementia and the decision-making process. *Geriatrics, 61*, 30–35.

Clay, R. A. (2006). Geropsychology grants in peril: Seven geropsychology training efforts have lost funding they receive through the Federal Graduate Psychology Education (GPE) Program. *Monitor on Psychology, 37* (4), 46.

Coleman, P. G. (1992). Personal adjustment in later life: Successful aging. *Reviews in Clinical Gerontology, 2*, 67–78.

Colenda, C. C., Bartels, S. C., & Gottlieb, G. L. (1999). The North American System of Care. In J. Copeland, M. Abou-Saleh, & D. Blazer (Eds.), *Principles and practices of geriatric psychiatry* (2nd ed., pp. 689–696). London: Wiley and Son.

Comas-Diaz, L., & Jacobsen, F. M. (1991). Ethnocultural transference and countertransference in the therapeutic dyad. *American Journal of Orthopsychiatry 61*, 392–402.

Connell, M., & Koocher, G. (2003). HIPAA & forensic practice. *American Psychology Law Society News, 23* (2), 16–19.

Constantinou, M., Ashendorf, L., & McCaffrey, R. J. (2002). When the 3rd party observer of a neuropsychological evaluation is an audio-recorder. *The Clinical Neuropsychologist, 16* (3), 407–412.

Constantinou, M., Ashendorf, L., & McCaffrey, R. J. (2005). Effects of a third party observer during neuropsychological assessment: When the observer is a video camera. *Journal of Forensic Neuropsychology, 4*, 39–48.

Cooper, J. (2007). Ethical caregiving in hard cases. *Annals of Long-Term Care, 15*, 25–27.

Cruzan v. Director, Missouri Department of Health, 497 US 261, 279 (1990).

Deidan, C., & Bush, S. (2002). Addressing perceived ethical violations by colleagues. In S. S. Bush & M. L. Drexler (Eds.), *Ethical issues in clinical neuropsychology* (pp. 281–305). Lisse, Netherlands: Swets & Zeitlinger Publishers.

DeLuca, J. (2005). Ethical challenges in geriatric neuropsychology, part I. In S. Bush (Ed.), *A casebook of ethical challenges in neuropsychology* (pp. 97–103). New York: Psychology Press.

Dickert, N., & Grady, C. (1999) What's the price of a research subject? Approaches to payment for research participation. *New England Journal of Medicine, 341*, 198–203.

Doukas, D. J., & McCollough, L. B. (1998). Assessing the values history of the elderly patient regarding critical and chronic care. In J. J. Gallo, W. Reichel, & L. Andersen (Eds.), *Handbook of geriatric assessment* (pp. 111–124). Rockville, MD: Aspen Publishers, Inc.

Eisenstadt v. Baird, 405 U.S. 438. (1972).

Eliopoulos, C. (1987). Ethical considerations. In C. Eliopoulos, *Gerontological nursing*, (2nd ed., pp. 401–406). Philadelphia: J. B. Lippincott Company.

Erikson E. H. (1982). *The life cycle completed: A review*. New York: Norton.

Erikson, E. H. (1963). *Childhood and society*. New York: Norton.

Erikson, E. H., Erikson, J. M., & Kivnick, H. Q. (1986). *Vital involvement in old age*. New York: Norton.

Federal Interagency Forum on Aging-Related Statistics. (2006). *Older Americans update 2006: Key indicators of well-being*. Retrieved December 28, 2007, from www.agingstats.gov/agingstatsdotnet/main site/default.aspx

Feinsod, F. M., & Wagner, C. (2007). 10 ethical principles in geriatrics and long-term care. *Annals of Long-Term Care, 15*, 24.

Fisher, C. B. (2003). Test data standard most notable change in new APA ethics code. *The National Psychologist*, Jan/Feb, 12–13.

Fisher, J. M., Johnson-Greene, D., & Barth, J. T. (2002). Examination, diagnosis, and interventions in clinical neuropsychology in general and with special populations: An overview. In S. Bush & M. Drexler (Eds.), *Ethical issues in clinical neuropsychology* (pp. 3–22). Lisse, Netherlands: Swets & Zeitlinger Publishers.

Fitting, M. D. (1986). Ethical dilemmas in counseling elderly adults. *Journal of Counseling & Development, 64*, 325–327.

Fletcher-Janzen, E., Strickland, L., & Reynolds, C. (Eds). (2000). *Handbook of cross-cultural neuropsychology*. New York: Kluwer Academic/Plenum Publishers.

Folstein, M. F., Folstein, S. E., & McHugh, P. R. (2002). *Mini-Mental State Examination*. Lutz, FL: Psychological Assessment Resources, Inc.

Friedland, B. (1994). Physician-patient confidentiality: Time to re-examine a venerable concept in light of contemporary society and advances in medicine. *Journal of Legal Medicine, 15*, 249–277.

Gavett, B. E., Lynch, J. K., & McCaffrey, R. J. (2005). Third party observers: The effect size is greater than you might think. *Journal of Forensic Neuropsychology, 4*, 49–64.

Gerontological Society of America, Task Force on Minority Issues in Gerontology. (1994). *Minority elders: Five goals toward building a public policy base*. Washington, DC: Author.

Gibson, W. T., & Pope, K. S. (1993). The ethics of counseling: A national survey of certified counselors. *Journal of Counseling & Development, 71*, 330–336.

Gostin, L. O. (2003). The judicial dismantling of the Americans with Disabilities Act. *Hastings Center Report, 33*(2), 9–11.

Grady, C. (2001). Money for research participation: does it jeopardize informed consent? *American Journal of Bioethics, 1*, 40–44.

Griswold v. Connecticut, 381 U.S. 479. (1965).

Haas, L., & Malouf, J. (2002). *Keeping up the good work: A practitioner's guide to mental health ethics* (3rd ed.). Sarasota, FL: Professional Resource Press.

Haber, C. (2004). Life extension and history: The continual search for the fountain of youth. *The Journals of Gerontology Series A: Biological Sciences and Medical Sciences, 59*, B515–B522.

Halpern, S. D. (2005). Towards evidence based bioethics. *British Medical Journal, 331*, 901–903.

Halpern, S. D., Karlawish, J. H. T., Casarett, D., Berlin, J. A., & Asch, D. A. (2004). Empirical assessment of whether moderate payments are undue or unjust inducements for participation in clinical trials. *Archives of Internal Medicine, 164*, 801–803.

Handelsman, M., Knapp, S., & Gottlieb, M. (2002). Positive ethics. In R. Snyder & S. Lopez (Eds.), *Handbook of positive psychology* (pp. 731–744). New York: Oxford University Press.

Hanson, S., Kerkhoff, T., & Bush, S. (2005). *Health care ethics for psychologists: A casebook*. Washington, DC: American Psychological Association.

Haut, M. W., & Muehleman, T. (1986). Informed consent: The effects of clarity and specificity on disclosure in a clinical interview. *Psychotherapy, 23*, 93–101.

Hawaii Psychiatric Society v. Ariyoshi, 481 F. Supp. 1028. (D. Hawaii, 1979).

Hays, J. R. (1999). Ethics of treatment in geropsychology: Status and challenges.

In M. Duffy (Ed.), *Handbook of counseling and psychotherapy with older adults* (pp. 662–676). New York: John Wiley & Sons.

He, W., Sengupta, M., Velkoff, V. A., DeBarros, K. A. (U.S. Census Bureau), (2005). *65+ in the United States: 2005. Current population reports, P23–209.* Washington, DC: U.S. Government Printing Office.

Health Care Financing Administration. (1992). Medicare and Medicaid programs: Preadmission screening and annual resident review. *Federal Register, 57,* 56450–56504.

Heaton, R. K., Miller, S. W., Taylor, M. J., & Grant, I. (2004). *Norms for an expanded Halstead-Reitan battery: Demographically adjusted neuropsychological norms for African American and Caucasian adults.* Lutz, FL: Psychological Assessment Resources.

High, D. M. (1994). Surrogate decision making: Who will make decisions for me when I can't? In G. A. Sachs & C. K. Cassel (guest editors), *Clinics in geriatric medicine: Clinical ethics* (pp. 445–462). Philadelphia: W. B. Saunders Company.

Hinrichsen, G. A. (2006). Why multicultural issues matter for practitioners working with older adults. *Professional Psychology: Research and Practice, 37,* 29–35.

Hofmann, M., Hock, C., Kuhler, A., & Muller-Spahn, F. (1996). Interactive computer-based cognitive training in patients with Alzheimer's disease. *Journal of Psychiatric Research, 30,* 493–501.

Holstein, M., & McCurdy, D. (1999). Ethical issues in mental health care. In T. F. Johnson (Ed.), *Handbook on ethical issues in aging* (pp. 165–186). London: Greenwood Press.

Iverson, G. L., & Slick, D. J. (2003). Ethical issues associated with psychological and neuropsychological assessment of persons from different cultural and linguistic backgrounds. In I. Z. Schultz & D. O. Brady (Eds.), *Psychological injuries at trial* (pp. 2066–2085). Chicago: American Bar Association.

Johnson-Greene, D. (2005). Ethical challenges in geriatric neuropsychology, part I. In S. Bush (Ed.), *A casebook of ethical challenges in neuropsychology* (pp. 104–110). New York: Psychology Press.

Kaplan, G. A., & Strawbridge, W. J. (1994). Behavioral and social factors in healthy aging. In R. P. Abeles, H. C. Gift, & M. G. Ory (Eds.), *Aging and quality of life* (pp. 57–78). New York: Springer Publishing.

Kehrer, C., Sanchez, P., Habif, U., Rosenbaum, J. G., & Townes, B. (2000). Effects of a significant-other observer on neuropsychological test performance. *The Clinical Neuropsychologist, 14,* 67–71.

Kim, S. Y. H. (2004). Evidence-based ethics for neurology and psychiatry research. *NeuroRx, 1,* 372–377.

Kitchener, K. S. (1984). Intuition, critical evaluation and ethical principles: The foundations for ethical decisions in counseling psychology. *The Counseling Psychologist, 12,* 43–55.

Kitchener, K. S. (2000). *Foundations of ethical practice, research, and teaching.* Mahwah, NJ: Erlbaum.

Knapp, S., & Vandecreek, L. (2003). *A guide to the 2002 revision of the American Psychological Association's Ethics Code.* Sarasota, FL: Professional Resource Press.

Knapp, S., & Vandecreek, L. (2004). A principle-based analysis of the 2002 American Psychological Association ethics code. *Psychotherapy: Theory, Research, Practice, Training, 41* (3), 247–254.

Knapp, S., & VandeCreek, L. (2006). *Practical ethics for psychologists: A positive approach.* Washington, DC: American Psychological Association.

Knight, B. G. (2004). *Psychotherapy with older adults* (3rd ed.). Thousand Oaks, CA: SAGE Publications.

Knight, B. G., & Satre, D. D. (1999). Cognitive behavioral psychotherapy with older adults. *Clinical Psychology: Science and Practice, 6,* 188–203.

Koocher, G. P., & Keith-Spiegel, P. (1998). *Ethics in psychology: Professional standards and cases* (2nd ed.). New York: Oxford University Press.

Kremer, T. G., & Gesten, E. L. (1998). Confidentiality limits of managed care and clients' willingness to self-disclose. *Professional Psychology: Research and Practice, 29,* 553–558.

Lebowitz, B. D., Pearson, J. L., Schneider, L. S., Reynolds, C. F., 3rd, Alexopoulos, G. S., Bruce, M. L., et al. (1997). Diagnosis and treatment of depression in late life. Consensus statement update. *Journal of the American Medical Association, 278* (14), 1186–1190.

Lichtenberg, P. A., & Hartman-Stein, P. E. (1997). Effective geropsychology practice in nursing homes. In L. VandeCreek, S. Knapp, & T. L. Jackson (Eds.), *Innovations in clinical practice: A source book* (pp. 265–281). Sarasota, FL: Professional Resource Press.

Lichtenberg, P. A., Smith, M., Frazer, D., Molinari, V., Rosowsky, E., Crose, R., Stillwell, N., et al. (1998). Standards for psychological services in long-term care facilities. *The Gerontologist, 38,* 122–127.

Lucas, J. A., Ivnik, R. J., Willis, F. B., Ferman, T. J., Smith, G. E., Parfitt, F. C., et al. (2005). Mayo's Older African Americans Normative Studies: Normative data for commonly used clinical neuropsychological measures. *The Clinical Neuropsychologist, 19,* 162–183.

Lynch, J. K. (2005). Effect of a third party observer on neuropsychological test performance following closed head injury. *Journal of Forensic Neuropsychology, 4,* 17–26.

Macciocchi, S. N., & Stringer, A. Y. (2002). Assessing risk and harm: The convergence of ethical and empirical considerations. *Archives of Physical Medicine & Rehabilitation, 82* (Suppl. 2), S15–S19.

Macklin, R. (1981). "Due" and "undue" inducements: On paying money to research subjects. *IRB: A Review of Human Subjects Research, 3,* 1–6.

Mahowald, M. B. (1994). So many ways to think: An overview of approaches to ethical issues in geriatrics. In G. A. Sachs & C. K. Cassel (guest editors), *Clinics in geriatric medicine: Clinical ethics* (pp. 403–418). Philadelphia, PA: W. B. Saunders Company.

McCaffrey, R. J. (guest editor), (2005). Third party observers. *Journal of Forensic Neuropsychology, 4* (2), Special Issue.

McCaffrey, R. J., Lynch, J. K., & Yantz, C. L. (2005). Third party observers: Why all the fuss? *Journal of Forensic Neuropsychology, 4,* 1–16.

McGee, G. (1997). Subject to payment? *Journal of the American Medical Association, 278,* 199–200.

McNeil, P. (1997). Paying people to participate in research. *Bioethics, 11,* 390–396.

McSweeny, A. J. (2005). Ethical challenges in geriatric neuropsychology, part I. In S. Bush (Ed.), *A casebook of ethical challenges in neuropsychology* (pp. 147–152). New York: Psychology Press.

Merriam-Webster. (1988). *Webster's 9th New Collegiate Dictionary.* Springfield, MA: Merriam-Webster, Inc.

Miles, T. P. (Ed.). (1999). *Full-color aging: Facts, goals, and recommendations for America's diverse elders.* Washington, DC: Gerontological Society of America.

Miller, D. J., & Thelen, M. H. (1986). Knowledge and beliefs about confidentiality in psychotherapy. *Professional Psychology: Research and Practice, 17,* 15–19.

Moore, S., Sandman, C. A., McGrady, K., & Kesslak, J. P. (2001). Memory training improves cognitive ability in patients with dementia. *Neuropsychological Rehabilitation, 11 (3/4),* 245–261.

Morgan, J. (2002). Ethical issues in the practice of geriatric neuropsychology. In S. S. Bush & M. L. Drexler (Eds.), *Ethical issues in clinical neuropsychology* (pp. 87–101). Lisse, NL: Swets & Zeitlinger Publishers.

Morgan, J. (2005). Ethical challenges in geriatric neuropsychology, part II. In S. Bush (Ed.), *A casebook of ethical challenges in neuropsychology* (pp. 153–158). New York: Psychology Press.

Myers, J. E. (1992). Wellness, prevention, development: The cornerstone of the profession. *Journal of Counseling and Development, 71,* 136–139.

Myers, J. E. (1999). Adjusting to role loss and leisure in later life. In M. Duffy (Ed.), *Handbook of counseling and psychotherapy with older adults* (pp. 41–56). New York: John Wiley & Sons.

National Association of Social Workers. (1999). *Code of ethics.* Retrieved September 1, 2007, from www.socialworkers.org/pubs/code/default.asp

National Association of Social Workers. (2006a). *Assuring the sufficiency of a frontline workforce. A national study of licensed social workers - special report: Social work services for older adults.* Retrieved September 9, 2007, from http://workforce.socialworkers.org/studies/aging/NASW_06_Aging.pdf.

National Association of Social Workers. (2006b). *Older Americans Act Amendments of 2006, Comments of National Association of Social Workers (NASW), submitted to Senate Health, Labor, Education and Pensions Committee.* Retrieved September 1, 2007, from www.naswdc.org/advocacy/letters/2006/062806Older.asp

National Board for Certified Counselors. (2005). *Code of ethics.* Retrieved April 22, 2008, from www.nbcc.org/ethics2

Nell, V. (2000). *Cross-cultural neuropsychological assessment: Theory and practice.* Mahway, New Jersey: Lawrence Erlbaum Associates.

Norris, M. P., Molinari, V., & Ogland-Hand, S. (Eds.). (2002). *Emerging trends in psychological practice in long-term care.* Binghamton, NY: Haworth Press.

Nowell, D., & Spruill, J. (1993). If it's not absolutely confidential, will information be disclosed? *Professional Psychology: Research and Practice, 24,* 367–369.

Olmstead v. L. C., 527 U.S. 581 (1999). Retrieved January 5, 2008, from www.accessiblesociety.org/topics/ada/olmsteadoverview.htm

Omnibus Budget Reconciliation Act of 1987, Pub. L. No. 100–203. Retrieved January 5, 2008, from www.ssa.gov/OP_Home/comp2/F100–203.html

Patient Self-Determination Act, Pub. L. No. 101–508 (1991).

Pinkston, J. B. (2005). Ethical challenges in geriatric neuropsychology, part I. In S. Bush (Ed.), *A casebook of ethical challenges in neuropsychology* (pp. 65–70). New York: Psychology Press.

Pinquart, M., & Soerensen, S. (2001). How effective are psychotherapeutic and other psychosocial interventions with older adults? A meta analysis. *Journal of Mental Health and Aging, 7*, 207–243.

Pope, K. S., & Vasquez, M. (2005). *How to survive and thrive as a therapist: Information, ideas, and resources for psychologists in practice*. Washington, DC: American Psychological Association.

Pope, K. S., & Vetter, V. A. (1992). Ethical dilemmas encountered by members of the American Psychological Association: A national survey. *American Psychologist, 47*, 397–411.

Pope, K. S., Tabachnick, B. G., & Keith-Spiegel, P. (1987). Ethics of practice: The beliefs and behaviors of psychologists as therapists. *American Psychologist, 42*, 993–1006.

Post, S. G. (2004). Establishing an appropriate ethical framework: The moral conversation around the goal of prolongevity. *The Journals of Gerontology Series A: Biological Sciences and Medical Sciences, 59*, B534–B539.

Rai, G. S. (Ed.). (1999). *Medical ethics and the elderly: Practical guide*. London: Informa Healthcare.

Redlich, F. C., & Pope, K. S. (1980). Ethics of mental health training. *Journal of Nervous and Mental Disease, 168*, 709–7 14.

Rehabilitation Act of 1973, Public Law 93–112.

Rehabilitation Act Amendments of 1992, Public Law 102–559.

Reichman, W., Coyne, A., Borson, S., Negrón, A. E., Rovner, B. W., Pelchat, R. J., Sakauye, K. M., Katz, P., Cantillon, M., Hamer, R. M. (1998). Psychiatric consultation in the nursing home: A survey of six states. *American Journal of Geriatric Psychiatry, 6*, 320–327.

Reichman, W. E., Streim, J. E., & Loebel, J. P. (2004). Legal, ethical, and policy issues. In D. G. Blazer, D. C. Steffens, & E. W. Busse (Eds.), *Textbook of geriatric psychiatry* (3rd ed., pp. 515–528). Washington, DC: American Psychiatric Publishing, Inc.

Reger, M. A., & Welsh, R. K. (2004). The relationship between neuropsychological functioning and driving ability in dementia: A meta-analysis. *Neuropsychology, 18*, 85–93.

Roe v. Wade, 410 U.S. 113. (1973).

Rosen, A. L. (2005). *Testimony to the Policy Committee of the White House Conference on Aging. The shortage of an adequately trained geriatric mental health workforce*. Retrieved March 16, 2008, from www.whcoa.gov/about/policy/meetings/Jan_24/Rosen%20WHCOA%20testimony.pdf

Ross, W. D. (1930/1998). What makes right acts right? In J. Rachels (Ed.), *Ethical theory* (pp. 265–285). New York: Oxford University Press. (Original work published 1930.)

Sachs, G. A., & Cassel, C. K. (Eds.). (1994). *Clinics in geriatric medicine: Clinical ethics*. Philadelphia: W. B. Saunders Company.

Samuda, R. J. (1998). *Psychological testing of American minorities: Issues and consequences* (2nd ed.). Thousand Oaks, CA: Sage Publications.

Sandoval, J., Frisby, C. L., Geisinger, K. F., Scheuneman, J. D. & Grenier, J. R. (Eds.). (1998). *Test interpretation and diversity: Achieving equity in assessment*. Washington DC: American Psychological Association.

Schatz, P. (2005). Ethical challenges with the use of information technology and telecommunications in neuropsychology, Part II. In S. S. Bush (Ed.), *A casebook of ethical challenges in neuropsychology* (190–198). New York: Psychology Press.

Scogin, F. (2003). *Depression and suicide in older adults resource guide*. Retrieved May 28, 2004, from http://www.apa.org/pi/aging/depression.html

Scogin, F. (section editor). (2007). Special section: Evidence-based psychological treatments of older adults. *Psychology and Aging, 22,* 1–55.

Smith-Bell, M., & Winslade, W. J. (1999). Privacy, confidentiality, and privilege in psychotherapeutic relationships. In D. N. Bersoff (Ed.), *Ethical conflicts in psychology* (2nd ed., pp. 151–155). Washington, DC: American Psychological Association.

Swiercinsky, D. P. (2002). Ethical issues in neuropsychological rehabilitation. In S. Bush & M. Drexler (Eds.), *Ethical issues in clinical neuropsychology* (pp. 135–163). Lisse, Netherlands: Swets & Zeitlinger.

Tarasoff v. Regents of the University of California, 551 P.2d 334 (Cal. 1976).

Taube, D. O., & Elwork, A. (1990). Researching the effects of confidentiality law on patients' self-disclosures. *Professional Psychology: Research and Practice, 2,* 72–75.

U.S. Department of Health and Human Services. (1999). Older adults and mental health. In *Mental health: A report of the Surgeon General*. Bethesda, MD: National Institute of Mental Health (pp. 335–401). Retrieved January 5, 2008, from www.surgeongeneral.gov/library/mentalhealth/pdfs/c5.pdf

U.S. Department of Health and Human Services. (2003). *Public Law 104–191: Health Insurance Portability and Accountability Act of 1996*. Retrieved November 24, 2008, from www.hhs.gov/ocr/hipaa

U.S. Department of Health and Human Services, Administration on Aging. (2006). *Public Law 109–365: Older Americans Act Amendments of 2006*. Retrieved January 5, 2008, from www.aoa.gov/oaa2006/Main_Site/oaa/oaa_full.asp

U.S. Department of Health and Human Services, Office of the Inspector General. (2001). *Medicare payments for psychiatric services in nursing homes: A follow-up* (DHHS Publ No OEI-02–99–00140). Retrieved January 5, 2008, from http://oig.hhs.gov/oei/reports/oei-02–99–00140.pdf.

United States ex rel. Friedrich LU v. David W. OU, et al. (03–3481) 368 F.3D 773, USCA 02–C-0072 (2004). Retrieved May 2, 2008, from caselaw.lp.findlaw.com/data2/circs/7th/033481p.pdf.

Vermont Agency of Natural Resources v. United States ex rel. Stevens (98–1828) 529 U.S. 765, 162 F.3d 195, reversed (2000). Retrieved May 2, 2008, from www.law.cornell.edu/supct/html/98–1828.ZO.html

Viens, A. M. (2001). Socio-economic status and inducement to participate. *American Journal of Bioethics, 1* (2), 1f–2f.

Washington v. Glucksberg, 117 SC 2258, 2270 (1997).

Waters, E. B., & Goodman, J. (1990). *Empowering older adults: Practical strategies for counselors*. San Francisco: Jossey-Bass.

Whalen v. Roe, 429 U.S. 589. (1976).

Wicclair, M. R. (1993). *Ethics and the elderly*. New York: Oxford University Press.

Wilde, E. A. (2005). Ethical challenges in geriatric neuropsychology, part I. In S. Bush (Ed.), *A casebook of ethical challenges in neuropsychology* (pp. 147–152). New York: Psychology Press.

Wilde, E. A., Bush, S., & Zeifert, P. (2002). Ethical issues in neuropsychology in medical settings. In S. Bush & M. L. Drexler (Eds.), *Ethical issues in clinical neuropsychology*, (pp. 195–221). Lisse, Netherlands: Swets & Zeitlinger Publishers.

Wilkenson, M., & Moore, A. (1997). Inducement in research. *Bioethics, 11*, 373–389.

Williams, L. (2000). Long-term care after *Olmstead v. L.C.*: Will the potential of the ADA's integration mandate be achieved? *Journal of Contemporary Health Law Policy, 17*, 205–239.

Wilson, R. S., Mendes de Leon, C. F., Barnes, L. L., Schneider, J. A., Bienias, J. L., Evans, D. A., et al. (2002). Participation in cognitively stimulating activities and risk of incident Alzheimer disease. *Journal of the American Medical Association 287*, 742–748.

Woods, K. M., & McNamara, J. R. (1980). Confidentiality: Its effect on interviewee behavior. *Professional Psychology, 11*, 714–721.

Wulach, J. S. (1993). *Law & mental health professionals: New York*. Washington, DC: American Psychological Association.

Yantz, C. L., & McCaffrey, R. J. (2006). Effects of a supervisor's observation on memory test performance of the examinee: Third party observer effect confirmed. *Journal of Forensic Neuropsychology, 4*, 27–38.

Zur, O. (2005). *The HIPAA compliance kit: Understanding and applying the regulations in psychotherapeutic practice* (3rd ed.). New York: W. W. Norton & Company.

Index

Ethical issues, continued and expanded
empirical study of, 24
Ethical principles
and professional guidelines, 25
and standards, 12
Ethical Principles of Psychologists and
Code of Conduct, 28
Ethical requirements
and guidelines, discrepancies between,
17
with other practice guidelines,
coordination principles, 34–35
Ethical resources, value ratings, 34t
Ethics Code of the American
Psychological Association
(2002a), 127, 128
Ethnogeriatrics, subspecialty of, 123
Experienced and informed colleagues, 18

F
False Claims Act 1986/"Lincoln Law",
129
False risk management principles,
20–21
Fear of confidentiality infringement,
86
Federal Claims Act, 129n
Fidelity, 13
Formal justice, 13
Futility of treatment, 14

G
General beneficence, 13
Geriatric medicine and long-term care
ethical principles, 13–15
Geriatric mental health professionals, 7
addressing perceived ethical
misconduct of colleagues, 134
appropriate professional conduct, 17
cooperation with other professionals,
74
ethical and legal requirements
governing professional
conduct, 32–35
ethical concerns of, 37
ethical decision making, 34
ethical obligation (beneficence), 138
forensic (i.e., legal) referrals, 73
importance of possessing specialized
skills in treating, 110–11
institutional practice, 74–76

mandates in New York State, 26
moral principles, 13
professional guidelines, 16–18
refrain entering into multiple
relationships, 73
respecting autonomous decision
making of competent older
adults, 72
Geriatric mental health services, 6
aspects requiring considerable ethical
attention, 40t
careful discussion and clarification
with all involved parties, 92
competence, 62–63
impact of big business on clinical
practice, whether and how to
address, 137
patient behaviour, ethnic, cultural, and
linguistic factors, 122
salient ethical issues, 37
threats to confidentiality, examples,
85t
Geriatric neuropsychology, ethical issues,
38
Geriatric psychiatry, 64
Good risk management principles, 20

H
Health Insurance Portability and
Accountability Act of 1996
(HIPAA), 29, 87
forensic considerations, 87–89
Section 160.102(3), 87
HIPAA's *Privacy rule*, 87
Hippocratic Oath, 34–35
History of patients' values, 93
Human relations, 67–76

I
Identifying and utilizing ethical and legal
resources
assessment, 97–98
ethical decision making, 48–50
health promotion, 127–29
human relations, 69
privacy, confidentiality, and informed
consent, 79–80
professional competence, 59–60
serving special populations,
117–18
treatment, 107

Vulnerable Older Adults
Health Care Needs and Interventions
Patricia M. Burbank, DNSc, RN, Editor

"It has been said that one measure of a society is the care it provides to its most vulnerable members. By taking on this challenge, Burbank and her colleagues have opened the door to addressing the needs of the most vulnerable among our older population."
— **Mathy Mezey**, RN, EdD, FAAN

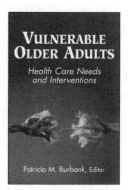

Based on the concept that vulnerability in the older populace encompasses those who are at increased risk for physical and psychosocial health problems, this book takes a closer look at vulnerability and how it affects five specific populations within the elderly: those incarcerated in prisons; the homeless; gay, lesbian, bisexual, and transgender people; those who are HIV positive or living with AIDS; and the frail.

Physical and psychosocial health care issues and needs are addressed as well as interventions and resources that can be implemented to care for these very specific populations and their requirements for successful physical and mental health care. The unique challenges of hospice care in prisons, the lack of services that cater to homeless older people, and the overall attitude towards helping elderly gay, lesbian, bisexual, or transgender people are some of the increasingly important issues covered.

Unique Features Include:
- Summary of the latest research and theoretical approaches to give health professionals a concise picture of health care needs of these older adult populations
- Interdisciplinary approach to care, cultural considerations, neglect, and abuse
- Discussion of strategies and resources for caring for older adults with dementia for each vulnerable population

2006 · 304pp · 978-0-8261-0208-9 · Hardcover

11 West 42nd Street, New York, NY 10036-8002 • Fax: 212-941-7842
Order Toll-Free: 877-687-7476 • Order Online: www.springerpub.com

SPRINGER PUBLISHING COMPANY

Aging and Disability

Crossing Network Lines

Michelle Putnam, PhD, Editor

There is a growing population at the intersection of aging and disability who increasingly rely on old community service systems for care—systems that currently cannot handle the increase in demand and the crossing of the care boundaries that have been set up between the aging and those with disability.

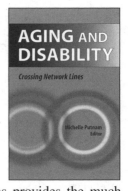

Michelle Putnam presents this volume to reflect the current research, facilitate collaboration across service networks, and encourage movement toward more effective service policies. Professional stakeholders evaluate the bridges and barriers to crossing network lines, and a chapter on current websites, agencies, and coalitions provides the much needed tools to bring collaboration into practice.

With contributions from those on the forefront of these issues, *Aging and Disability* will provide a basis for understanding why our aging and disability networks have so long been separated and what we can do to bridge that gap.

Partial Contents:

Section One: Introduction to Cross-Network Collaborations and Coalitions
  Moving from Separate to Crossing Aging and Disability Service Networks; Facilitators and Barriers to Crossing Network Lines

Section Two: Collaborations and Coalitions in Practice
  Building Intersystem Partnerships at the Intersection of Aging and Developmental Disabilities; Partnerships and Coalitions across Aging and Disability Service Networks

Section Three: Research toward Improving Services at the Intersections of Aging and Disability
  Stakeholder Involvement in Intervention, Research, and Evaluation; The Government-Wide Shift in Accountability for Results

2006 · 296pp · 978-0-8261-5565-8 · Hardcover

11 West 42nd Street, New York, NY 10036-8002 • Fax: 212-941-7842
Order Toll-Free: 877-687-7476 • Order Online: www.springerpub.com

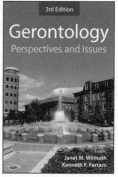

SPRINGER PUBLISHING COMPANY

Health Promotion and Aging

Fourth Edition

Practical Applications for Health Professionals

David Haber, PhD

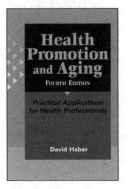

"...[this book] should be on the bookshelf of every student and every professor in any one of the health disciplines...[it] is a resource that pulls together everything that a health provider would need to know about promoting health and quality of life for older adults."
—From the Foreword by **Barbara Resnick**, PhD, FAAN

Continuing to advocate for health professionals becoming health educators and a more informed, healthier aging population, David Haber has updated this fourth edition with discussion and analysis of major issues and topics in the field, including:

- A critique of the MyPyramid Food Guide
- How to change medical encounters into health encounters
- Descriptions of model health programs
- A review of the 2006 Surgeon General's Report on secondhand smoke
- Critical analysis of Medicare Part D
- The benefits of pet support
- Life review and cognitive fitness
- Appraisals of complementary and alternative practices

Innovative ideas on public policy and aging, examples of stand-out community health advocacy, and a final chapter on the future of the field complete this integrated look at health, community, and aging.

2007 · 600pp · 978-0-8261-8463-4 · Hardcover

11 West 42nd Street, New York, NY 10036-8002 • Fax: 212-941-7842
Order Toll-Free: 877-687-7476 • Order Online: www.springerpub.com